every
BODY
YOGA

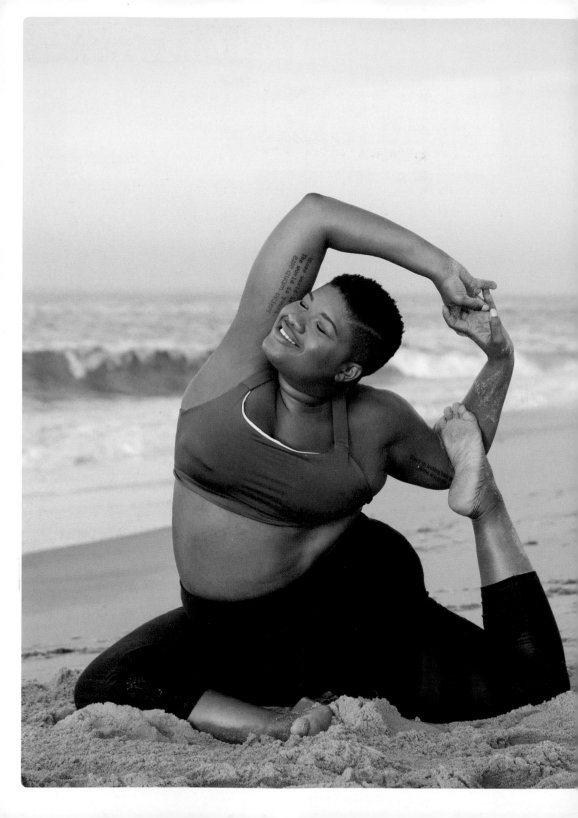

every
BODY
YOGA

LET GO OF FEAR,
GET ON THE MAT,
LOVE YOUR BODY.

JESSAMYN STANLEY

Workman Publishing • New York

Library of Congress Cataloging-in-Publication Data is available.

ISBN 978-0-7611-9311-1

Design by Becky Terhune
Yoga portraits by Christine Hewitt
Yoga postures by Jonathan Conklin
Cover photo by Hannah Khymych
Additional photo credit: Page 202 photo © Zoe Litaker
Yoga models: Jaclyn Atkinson, Laura Cabrera, Crissy Hastings, Charlie Radin
Hair and makeup by Stephanie Gomez
Special thanks to Jade Yoga

Workman books are available at special discounts when purchased in bulk for
premiums and sales promotions as well as for fund-raising or educational use.
Special editions or book excerpts can also be created to specification.
For details, contact the Special Sales Director at the address below,
or send an email to specialmarkets@workman.com.

Workman Publishing Co., Inc.
225 Varick Street
New York, NY 10014-4381
workman.com

WORKMAN is a registered trademark of Workman Publishing Co., Inc.

Printed in China
First printing February 2017

10 9 8 7 6 5 4 3 2 1

Every Body Yoga was written with the belief that absolutely anyone can build a
smart and safe yoga practice. However, if you have any concerns about yoga's
impact on your physical health, please consult a physician before attempting
any of the poses or sequences in the book. The publisher and author are not
liable for any complications, injuries, loss, or medical problems arising from
or in connection with using this book.

For Jesse "the Jet."
Because you've always believed in me—
even when I didn't believe in myself.

CONTENTS

WHY DID I WRITE THIS BOOK?

In the summer of 2012, I was an unemployed grad-school dropout and relatively new to yoga. I enjoyed going to classes, but like many other yoga students who look "different," I always left the studio feeling a vague sense of discrimination at the hands of my teachers and fellow students. I was also strapped for cash and could barely afford the occasional drop-in class. So I turned my focus to developing a home practice. I began photographing and documenting my yoga asana practice and posting the shots on Instagram. At the time, Instagram was a fairly new kind of social media, but there was already a small community of yoga teachers and practitioners who were using the app to share their home practices. I quickly found my place in this virtual community and with it, a sense of inclusion and encouragement that I'd never felt in any live yoga class.

That's when everything changed. I became ravenous for information beyond the physical poses I'd encountered in studio classes. I studied anatomy, the history of yoga, and the evolution of various yoga lineages. I got certified as a yoga instructor. Today, I have the incredible privilege to travel the world teaching the practice I love so much.

As much as social media has given me, it shouldn't be the only source of inspiration for people who don't fit the typical yoga mold. That's why

I wrote this book. Because all yoga bodies deserve to be represented in print, not just those that are slender, female, and white.

I wrote this book for every fat person, every old person, and every exceptionally short person. I wrote it for every person who has called themselves ugly and every person who can't accept their beauty. I wrote it for every person who is self-conscious about their body.

I wrote it for every human being who struggles to find happiness on a daily basis, and for anyone who has ever felt overwhelmed by the mere act of being alive. I've been there. We all have.

Yoga is for everybody and <u>EVERY</u> <u>BODY</u>. You don't have to be thin and you don't have to be fat. You don't have to be a specific color or commit to a specific diet. You don't have to earn (or have access to) a certain amount of money.

You don't have to embody anything other than your truest and most honest self in order to practice yoga.

You don't have to embody anything other than your truest and most honest self in order to practice yoga. You don't have to omit the sadness, the anger, and all of the other "ugly" emotions that flavor our lives.

You don't have to be anyone other than yourself.

And I think it's high time that someone shouted it loud enough so everyone can hear.

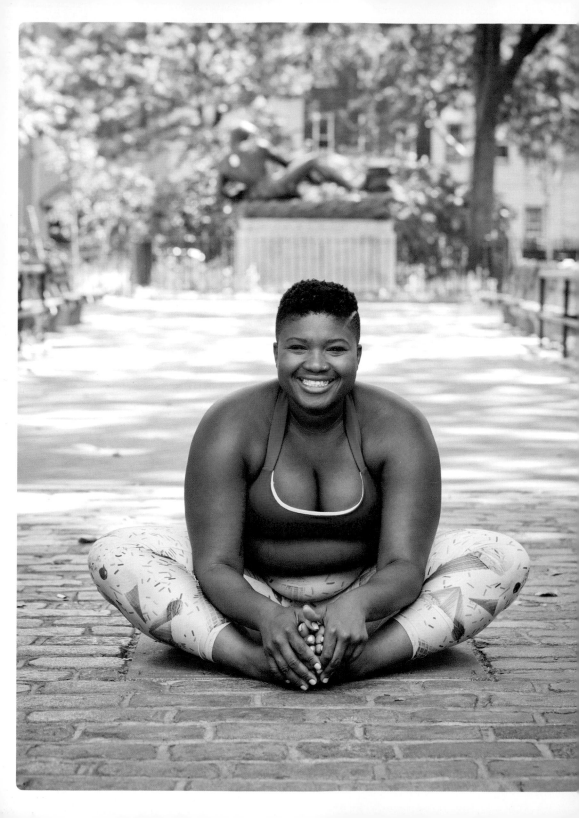

PART I
Let's Get Warmed Up

"HEY, JESSAMYN, HOW DO I START PRACTICING YOGA?"

Let's just say that if I had a nickel for every time someone has asked this question within my hearing/reading/breathing range over the past five years, I would be ballin' Bill Gates–style. Apparently, when you show the internet your fat ass in a yoga pose, everyone wants to know how the hell you managed to do it.

Usually, people ask me this question in situations where I couldn't possibly give an adequate response, like while I'm waiting for my date to finish using the bathroom at a friend of a friend's cocktail party, or while I'm at the grocery store after spending all day in line at the DMV. And even though I *want* to enter into a completely serene and helpful dialogue that starts with something along the lines of, "Oh my God, thank you for asking! Of course, I can *ABSOLUTELY* explain to you in thirty words or less every single bit of information you need to know in order to start practicing yoga," I'm not really serene and I don't have much of a poker face. My honest answer is just too vast and long-winded to be adequately summed up even in the most nightmarish DMV line, and I'm usually too overwhelmed to formulate an appropriate shorthand response. Therefore, I'm sure the look on my face betrays what I'm thinking, which is basically "HOW THE FUCK DO YOU THINK I COULD ACTUALLY ADEQUATELY ANSWER THIS QUESTION IN THE MIDDLE OF WHOLE FOODS

RIGHT NOW??" The question asker usually backs away slowly, leaving me standing there with the grimace of a gargoyle while the Whole Foods cashier tries to pretend they *didn't* just witness the world's most awkward human interaction.

If you and I have had this interaction, I apologize. I know you were just trying to get clarity on a topic that a lot of people seem to have questions about. It's probably why you (yes, YOU, the person reading these words right now) decided to flip through this book while hiding from your Tinder date in the back corner of Barnes & Noble. Or maybe you saw an Instagram picture of me turning my body upside down or bending my spine in a way that seems as though I should *definitely* see an exorcist and thought to yourself, "Damn, if that fat bitch can do it, I bet I can too!"

Perhaps you've tried yoga in the past and it proved to be an absolutely wretched experience. Maybe you've given up faith in the potential for your own yoga practice. Maybe you thought it was boring, or just WAY harder than you expected. Maybe you're thinking that you and I share some common ground that you've never been able to find with other yoga teachers. Because your takeaway from seeing a picture of me—a fat girl practicing yoga in her underwear—is that it can't be that hard. So maybe you can do what I can do. I mean, it'll probably take a little effort and sweat, but you'll be headstanding and deep backbending in no time, right?

Um, yeah . . . I think you are absolutely correct. I think that if you have body issues, or if you've got shit raging in your head about your body shape, size, or condition, particularly as it pertains to yoga, then I *do* think you can learn a lot from my experience. Because you're totally right: I *am* fat. I am *not* the person you would typically imagine teaching or practicing yoga. Or even sitting behind a *reception desk* in a yoga studio. I know how it feels to be an outsider. I know how it feels to be discouraged and excluded in an environment that's meant to foster calm and serenity.

The truth is that you only need to attend one drop-in class at your local yoga studio to notice that the modern Western yoga world is very diverse and practitioners come in every color, shape, and size in the flesh-toned rainbow. But if you're only paying attention to the *media's* idea of a yoga practitioner—one that mirrors the stereotypical image of physician-approved Western health: slender, long, and young—it's easy to see how you might feel a little alienated and lost.

This may be an anticlimactic proclamation, but I was once just as alienated and lost as you're feeling right now. When I found yoga, I was completely buried under the melodramatic woes of my life. I was emotionally damaged—love, loss, and the realities of life had battered my heart and constructed complex walls around the core of my spirit—and I'd been trapped under body issues basically since exiting the womb.

My practice helps me transcend the all-consuming nonsense of daily life.

I grew up in a predominantly white Southern suburban community—and I was the epitome of a big, black, and beautiful African queen trapped in a sea of dainty-lipped, pale-skinned sea nymphs. I found it nearly impossible to reconcile my Afro-American natural beauty with the one-dimensional (and very, very white) portrayals of beauty that surrounded me. As a preteen, I needed constant reassurance of my beauty and, as time went on, I grew to loathe my naturally thick and kinky hair. Though I was always the fattest, the slowest, and the least athletic, I idolized the stereotypical beauty of cheerleaders. Despite my complete lack of natural flexibility and balance, I tried to join my middle school cheerleading team. A few years later, I became obsessed with losing weight. Harboring sustained hatred for your body? Yeah, it isn't a good look. And I don't think it's a stretch to say that my childhood self-hatred created some very nasty, adult-size emotional wounds. In retrospect, all of these experiences directly point to a need for *some* kind of yoga. And *not* as an exercise routine, but as a way to stop acting like my own worst enemy. It only took me the greater portion of three decades to figure that out.

My practice helps me transcend the all-consuming nonsense of daily life. It allows me to step outside of my mundane fears, endless obsessions, and senseless anger. I don't know about you, but I've never had that kind of feeling from other kinds of physical exercise. And it's because yoga is NOT just exercise—it's a life path. And if you allow it, the yogic path will envelop every moment of your life—every breath, every interaction, every gaze, and every thought.

You see, when Westerners talk about "yoga," they are almost invariably talking about "asana,"[1] otherwise known as the fancy, gymnastics-esque postures that someone in your state is probably teaching at this exact moment. However, asana is only one limb of an eight-limbed path, and true yoga practitioners align their lives in pursuit of fulfilling all eight limbs, not just asana—important things like breathing, discipline, concentration, meditation. (I go into this more on page 35.)

The eight-limbed path of yoga can help answer the questions we spend our entire lives obsessing over. Not superficial questions: Am I fat? Am I pretty? or Will I get that job? I'm talking about REAL questions, deeper questions, the ones that get embedded in our psyches during childhood, the questions that continue to fester during adolescence, bloom during adulthood, and continue to haunt us: What is my worth? Do I deserve love? What is my purpose? What if my dreams don't come true?

Even if you're an anti–New Age, dyed-in-the-wool fitness buff, a person with absolutely no interest in the "spiritual" side of yoga, someone who gives zero fucks about the eight-limbed path and never will, I don't think you're immune to the real power of yoga. Because I don't care how "together" your shit is, we're *all* looking for answers, for balance, for peace.

My life madness certainly didn't end once I started practicing yoga. But no matter the circumstances, my practice has been there for me—even when I couldn't find a way to crawl off the ground, when I thought self-hate and self-loathing would be the end of me, my yoga practice helps me accept the fact that bad judgment and big missteps are the toll we pay for being present in our lives. Ultimately, yoga has made me realize that happiness doesn't come when we magically become *better* people. The practice is a reminder that we deserve to be happy today, in this exact moment, because we are *already* absolutely perfect.

---

1 Asana = pose = posture. I tend to use these words interchangeably to describe yoga poses.

UM, YOU STILL HAVEN'T ANSWERED MY QUESTION

Okay. So how do you start practicing yoga? This book is my answer.

I'm going to give you a crash course in yoga—I like to think of it as "Yoga 101"—where I break down the basics of modern yogic history, the core elements of the eight-limbed path, and various Modern yoga styles as well as all the tools and supplies that will light up your own practice. I'll answer questions asked by (literally) every beginner yoga student. And I'll teach you your ABCs—my favorite key yoga poses. These are the poses that formed the bedrock of my yoga practice when I began practicing, and which I still vary and flow together to this day. By establishing a strong connection with all of these poses, you'll develop a firm foundation of yoga asana, knowledge that you can take with you into any yoga studio in the world.

Then I'll help you put it all together with a series of yoga sequences tailored to specific moods and emotional needs. The beautiful yoga practitioners featured in the book—Laura, Chrissie, Charlie, Jaclyn—are all trained yoga teachers who don't necessarily fit the stereotypical yoga teacher mold. Just like me. Just like you. Don't be surprised. There are more of us than you might think.

I believe that the truest way any of us can be inspired to practice yoga is by hearing the true life stories of our fellow practitioners and teachers. These uniquely personal life sagas—stories full of more heartache, injury, addiction, loss, and skin-crawling moments than a soap opera—motivate us along the yogic path. So, if you'll indulge me, I'm going to tell you a few stories from my own life. Because I'm no angel, and I've sure as hell made mistakes. And, let's face it, we both know you've fallen on your ass a time or two. From friend to friend, take comfort in knowing that I am your lifelong comrade in arms.

"IS THIS A CULT?"

My first yoga experience was hell on earth. Are you hearing me? HELL. ON. EARTH.

I was sixteen when my aunt Tracy dragged me to a Bikram yoga class. My mother's youngest sister, Tracy Baldwin, was the epitome of glamour for teenaged Jessamyn—the "jet-setting inspirational career woman" of my genesis. She was as tall as an Amazon and startlingly beautiful, with a cutting wit and a sense of humor as dry as rye toast; a world traveler who always returned home with wild stories that were just salacious enough to send her niece into a tailspin of daydreams. My auntie had been engaged on several different occasions, but she'd never walked down the aisle, and she wore her unmarried, child-free status as a badge of honor. She devoted a portion of every summer to shepherding me, my younger brother, and all of our cousins through the travails of early adolescence. Aunt Tracy was the woman who taught me how to Nair my upper lip hair. She was especially helpful when it came to learning the ins and outs of using one's sexuality to confuse and confound men, and when it came to verbally bitch slapping a playground adversary, she was a language arsenal.

That fateful summer, my world-wise auntie was obsessed with Bikram yoga, and she encouraged me to join her at a class. For those of you who have never tried it, Bikram is a series of twenty-six yoga postures performed over ninety minutes in a very hot room. How hot is very hot? Roughly 105 degrees. And when you're a whiny, chubby high school student trapped in a sweaty and stiflingly hot yoga studio instead of camping out on your aunt's couch watching her endless supply of VHS tapes, one ninety-minute yoga session can quickly turn into a nightmare.

In a room full of advanced middle-aged practitioners, I was a fat teenage novice, and I stuck out like a sore thumb. The teacher clearly had doubts about my ability to survive the class, and I did too. The heat of the room was completely unreasonable. I couldn't fathom how red-blooded human beings were actually expected to survive an entire hour and a half without even a puff of air-conditioning. Also, the studio's smell was overwhelming. Sweat and wall-to-wall carpeting don't mix, but it was clear from the moment I rolled out my mat that absolutely no one in the room cared about such things.

I wanted to duck out of the class before we'd even finished the opening rounds of pranayama, or breath work. In any Bikram yoga class in the world, you will encounter the intense dual rounds of nasal inhales and oral exhales that bookend the yoga sequence. The Bikram pranayama is particularly killer, even for experienced practitioners. The other students in the class were breathing so hard, deep, and loud that they looked like they were trying to impersonate a colony of dragons. I thought I might see smoke come out of at least one person's nostrils. How could something as utterly basic and *human* as breathing be so goddamn hard? I'd been doing it all my life, and yet I found these breathing exercises to be impossible.

I was a fat teenage novice, and I stuck out like a sore thumb.

The balance postures were similarly difficult, and not just because of my naturally clumsy nature. Thanks to the relentless heat, I was sweating like a pig on a New York City subway platform in August. Sweat was pouring from every possible orifice. My kneecaps were sweating. The backs of my elbows were sweating. There was condensation on my fucking toe hair. And in spite of the towel I'd been advised to drape over my mat, the sweat made it nearly impossible to stand up straight, let alone grab my foot behind my head or any of the other inscrutable shenanigans my classmates seemed to be doing so effortlessly.

About a third of the way into the class, I became convinced that my death by heat exhaustion was imminent. I had to get out of there. With my dignity dripping off my finger webbing, I managed to crawl out of Satan's yoga sauna. The wave of AC-sodden oxygen that met me in the hallway was a relief on par only with manna from heaven. However, I soon learned why teachers discourage students from exiting hot studios mid-class: When a fatigued student reenters the stiflingly hot room from a relatively cold space, their internal temperature shift can be abrupt and painful, with disastrous results. Upon returning to my mat, I felt a wave of nausea unlike anything I'd ever experienced. I spent the rest of the class in a heap on my yoga mat, simultaneously trying not to cry and wanting to melt into the atmosphere. I'm not ashamed to say that I hated every one of those ninety minutes, and my Emmy award–worthy dramatics after class resulted in a round of restorative Cook Out milkshakes for both me and my aunt.[2] Yoga was *obviously* not for me.

HOW BAD COULD IT REALLY BE?

Seven years later, when my friend Anna asked me to join her for a class at our local Bikram yoga studio in Winston-Salem, North Carolina, my knee-jerk reaction was something along the lines of "You've gotta be fucking kidding me."

Anna is one of the bubbliest and most enthusiastic people I've ever known. I mean, this girl could simultaneously tap dance, sing, twirl a baton, and balance a checkbook, all with a smile. She worked hard to make me sip the Bikram Kool-Aid. "It's hard for everyone at first," she said cheerfully, encouraging me with the kind of comfortable, blissed-out tone that you can't get without at least a sliver of a meditation practice or a regular

---

2 It just occurred to me that most non–North Carolinians probably don't know about the time-tested calming effects of a cold Cook Out milkshake. All I can say is (in my best sorghum-glazed drawl), "There ain't one better." I recommend banana puddin' flavor. You're welcome.

marijuana-smoking regimen. "But I promise it will make you feel so good! And it's great exercise too!"

I couldn't deny that I could use the exercise. My habit of attending the occasional fitness class had slowed considerably since college and, in the wake of various romantic catastrophes, I had developed an intimate and comforting relationship with Taco Bell and Pizza Hut that made me feel sluggish even on my best days. I was depressed, and although I was actively looking for a way out of my emotional hole, I didn't see how yoga could possibly help.

But optimism grows in strange places, and before long I found myself softening to Anna's pleas. It didn't hurt that our local Bikram studio was promoting a discounted intro month class pass at the time, one of those really good deals that you hem and haw over until you just throw up your hands and say, "Well, how bad could it really be if I can attend an entire month of unlimited classes for only thirty dollars?" (There's also a distinct possibility that the reason I finally caved to the gravitational pull of Bikram yoga is because it's actually a cult and Anna had recruited me in the same way new cult members have been recruited for, legit, thousands of years.)

With my tail between my legs and my dad's old Pilates mat under my arm, I finally made my way to the Bikram studio on Fayette Street in early fall 2011. My memories from that first class are like odd whiffs of random scents. I remember feeling as though everyone's eyes were on me. And by "everyone" I mean every single living and breathing human, from the person casually walking out of the studio to the bored studio receptionist to the person who chose to roll out her mat as far away from me as possible. (In my self-sabotaging mind, it was NEVER because they simply wanted to practice in a different part of the room.[3]) Every single gaze felt like a

---

3 For the record, there are a million logistical reasons that go into selecting a mat spot in your typical Bikram yoga studio. No one likes to set up their mat in the farthest corner of the room, right next to the humidifier, in what's quite possibly the hottest part of the classroom. Well, no one except for yours truly, trying to hide myself as far away as possible from the teacher.

judgment. "What are YOU doing here?" the gazes said. "Your fat ass does not deserve to be here."

I truly believed that I was unfit to be in the yoga studio. But as the class gained momentum and we started practicing the asana, I eventually had to tell my mind to shut the hell up, and not for any other reason than the fact that it was SO HARD and I needed to focus my full attention on not collapsing. Nothing had changed in the years since my last yoga experience. I hadn't magically become stronger, and the poses hadn't magically become easier.

In fact, some of the poses completely knocked me off my feet, both emotionally and physically. Less than twenty minutes into class, the teacher told us to go into Chair Pose (page 82). First, you start by just planting your feet firmly on the ground, bending your knees, and sinking your hips back, your arms extended parallel to the ground. The second variation requires that you rise onto your tiptoes and repeat the same action. And in the third variation, you bend your knees while on your tippy toes, then cross one ankle over the opposite knee and then continue to bend the knees SO DEEPLY that your butt hovers about 6 to 8 inches above the ground. And as if that wasn't hard enough, you have to stare at yourself in a huge mirror.

Does it sound intense as fuck? THAT'S BECAUSE IT IS.

The Bikram ideology says that by gazing into your own eyes and using them as a point of balance, you are given the opportunity to see within the eyes of your one and only true teacher—yourself. But by this point in my life, I had grown accustomed to avoiding my own reflection if I thought I looked like shit. I mean, it's pretty common fat girl knowledge that we're not allowed to wear anything fun or interesting while working out. I always thought thin girls were the only people who were allowed to wear cute bralettes and tight leggings, so on that particular day, I had followed proper fat girl exercise apparel protocol by wearing my baggiest T-shirt and pairing it with my ugliest gym shorts. I associated so much shame with my body, I didn't think I deserved to wear clothing that actually made me feel good. The strength of truly toxic shame comes when it's allowed to fester, like an open wound. And, by the time I tried to look myself in the eye during this yoga class, my body shame had been festering for the better part of two decades. I still don't know why I didn't run screaming from the class. Sometimes I think I was in such a bad place that nothing I could feel in the hot-as-hell yoga studio could be worse than what I was feeling every other part of the day. So I didn't run from the class. I stayed to the bitter end. And I kept coming back.

It wasn't easy. The physical challenge of struggling through Chair Pose in a room full of huffing and puffing yoga dragons combined with the emotional intensity of all that eye contact caused me to swell with waves of anger and self-pity. This became a familiar pattern in the early days of my practice. When I found a pose difficult, I became defensive and prideful. Often, I *literally* stopped practicing until the next pose. My teachers and fellow practitioners saw a surly-looking, curvy black femme standing on her mat in stoic silence, grouchy because her body wouldn't bend the way her mind wanted. But on the inside, I was in tears. "Why can't I do it?" I thought. "What's wrong with me? Everyone around me is making this look so easy! WHY CAN THEY DO IT AND I CAN'T?"[4]

Eventually, the tears stopped flowing—I guess you can't cry forever, right?

The desire to cry inconsolably wasn't really what I expected from a practice that my friend had assured me would calm and relax my spirit. This sensation could be overwhelming to the point of debilitation. Some days it felt like the mother of all triumphs to just drag my ass into my car, drive it to the yoga studio, actually get *out* of the car, walk into the studio, and roll out my mat. But at some point I stopped fighting it. When my internal baby would rear up, instead of yelling at myself, I just let myself have a moment of being upset, and eventually, the tears stopped flowing—I guess you can't cry forever, right?

---

4 Have you ever felt this way before? Actually, forget it—I KNOW you've felt this way before. The thing is, I hear this all the time from new yoga students. When they approach a pose that's difficult for them, they get supremely pissed at themselves and the universe, thus beginning a landslide of negative self-talk and waking up a sleeping baby inside themselves that refuses to stop crying once its nap is interrupted. Well, trust me—I've been there. In a really intense way, and not just in the beginning of my practice. It happens to the best of us all the time.

Then, with big, imaginary, salt-cracked tear streaks on my cheeks, I'd ask myself if I had bothered to look in my eyes in the mirror during my failed attempt at the asana. More often than not the answer would be no. I would start to stare, but then I'd be distracted by the parts of myself that were not up to my personal standards—my quivering belly, my gelatinous arm fat, the fact that my chins wiggled even when I wasn't talking. It took a lot to ignore the parts of my body that I perceived as subpar—they felt like permanent reminders of my inadequacy.

But when I would let my gaze rest solely on my eyes in the mirror—actually dared to look within the eyes of my own "true" teacher—I saw what really stopped me from being able to find balance: Fear. I was afraid. Of what? Who knows. Probably my own potential greatness. But when I actually made eye contact with myself, when I caught and held my own gaze and carefully followed the alignment instructions offered by the teacher, I forced myself to stare down every dark thought I'd ever had about myself. And in the process, I was able to find a sense of comfort in the pose.

I was still aware that on many levels, my version of Chair Pose looked very different from my fellow practitioners. My alignment was sloppy and not as advanced as that of most of the people in the room. But when I would fall out of a pose, I would give myself the chance to try again. Without judgment or fear—after all, I'd already fallen out of the pose; why not just give it another try for fun? It's possible that I hadn't given myself the chance to *try* in such a carefree way since childhood. In fact, until that day on Fayette Street, it's possible that I'd never allowed myself the chance to trust myself. And that was a triumph all my own, a triumph I hadn't felt in years.

THE ELEPHANT IN THE ROOM

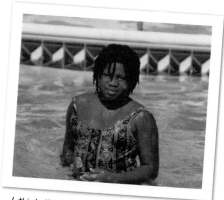

I think this photo adequately sums up how awkward I felt for the entirety of the 1990s.

Here's the thing: I'm fat. And I've always been fat. Well, maybe not always. I suppose most doctors would say I had every opportunity to be a normal, happy, thin kid. But instead I turned into a fat, occasionally smelly, supremely awkward weirdo. My mom has always blamed my early weight gain on the lunches served at my elementary and middle schools. She abhorred the chicken fingers, lasagna, and sloppy joes that my public schools dished out, chock-full of the toxic shit that's been making Americans fat for the past hundred years or so. But frankly, the food we ate at school wasn't all that different from the food I was eating at home.

I grew up in a traditional black Southern family. Holidays meant deep-fried turkeys, vats of pork-coated collard greens, lard-rich meat gravy, and plenty of fresh biscuits to soak up all the juices. My mother resented this gastronomical heritage with the fiery passion of a thousand suns. She saw what the traditional foods of our homeland had done to our family members, making diabetes and heart disease common among older and younger generations alike, and she wanted a different future for her family.

Tangela was part of the late-1980s wave of feminist mommies. These were college educated, post–second wave women who exhibited their love of their children by absorbing every bit of doctor-approved, nutrition-related gobbledygook available. My mommy denounced the ham-hock-drenched

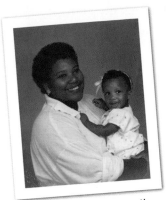

Tangela taught me to smile on command AND make kale smoothies for breakfast.

veggies and fatback-laden diets of her heritage. Our family was solidly working class, but she tried her best to mesh our meager food budget with the health ideals she read about in books and magazines. She was a devotee of Susan Powter, and was willing to try every new holistic dietary trend under the sun. Way before Jessica Seinfeld was sneaking spinach into brownies, Tangela had her eyes peeled for opportunities to trick us into eating the food she read about in her favorite hippie-dippy magazines and books. She had us drinking kale smoothies and eating chia seeds before they were on the radar of every healthy-living food blogger under the sun. She was all about echinacea and other green supplements, and her Jack LaLanne "Power Juicer" was one of her most prized possessions.[5]

Much to her chagrin, Tangela's baby daddy (also known as my loving father) was and continues to be a stone-cold macaroni and cheese and root beer aficionado. Jesse Stanley has always been a physical powerhouse—he was a celebrated athlete and bodybuilder in his youth, allowing him the metabolic freedom to eat whatever he pleased. Along with a tendency toward social introversion, my father passed his love of cheddar, noodles, and mountain soda brews to his children. And anyone who thinks that even the BEST kale smoothie can compare to even a single sip of crisp, ice-cold Barq's root beer is just kidding themselves. So despite our mother's best efforts, my brother Gabriel and I happily ate our way toward chubby bellies, plump thighs, and juicy neck rolls.

And if I'm really being honest, my fatness wasn't just the product of extra helpings of mac and

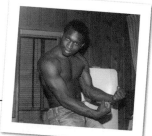

Jesse "the Jet" Stanley

---

5 To this day, Tangela still stays about that green life, though now she'll talk your ear off about her favorite gluten-free baking techniques over the deafening roar of her beloved Vitamix.

cheese on Thanksgiving or the quintessential Stanley family special-occasion Golden Corral buffet pig-outs.[6] No, just like a lot of true food addicts, my complicated relationship to food was born out of a place of sadness, not celebration.

Back in 1995, shortly after she returned home from an epic voyage to the Fourth World Conference on Women in Beijing, my mom became very sick. I mean, *really* sick. I was eight years old. At first, it didn't seem like that big of a deal. Kind of like a really bad cold, you know? But the cold just kept getting progressively worse. And eventually my mom's body started retaining excess water. Like, *a lot* of excess water. She started to swell up like Violet Beauregarde in *Charlie and the Chocolate Factory*. Eventually, she was almost completely bedridden—her body was congested with all kinds of fluids, and she was constantly coughing up chunky streams of brown, yellow, and green. My parents sought out all kinds of medical specialists, but she was continuously misdiagnosed. Our lives starting moving to the morose rhythm that only sickness and sadness can orchestrate.

Due to my mother's mounting medical bills and his status as our family's sole breadwinner, my beloved papa bear was forced to work round the clock to keep our little nuclear family afloat. Responsibility in hand, Jesse spent the first two decades of my life pulling night and day shifts at two different jobs. In fact, most of my strongest childhood memories of my dad are of stolen moments early in the morning and late at night when he would have an odd hour between shifts. He always made time to answer homework questions or listen to my complaints or fears about enemies and various obstacles, but, understandably, the few hours of his day not logged on an employee time clock needed to be spent in a state of sleep and energy restoration. And because my mom was basically bedridden for the majority of late 1995 through early 1998, my brother

---

6 Golden Corral was my favorite restaurant as a child—we were never wealthy enough to regularly dine out, but any time there was an opportunity for a special-occasion restaurant meal, I would always submit a request for the buffet at Golden Corral. Even to this day, my mother absolutely loathes Golden Corral—she still (un)affectionately calls it "The Trough."

and I would comfort each other by watching VHS tapes of musicals and eating everything under the sun.[7]

I'm sure my mom would love to think we were making ourselves brown rice pilaf and kale chips while she was out of commission, but that was *so* not the case. We were kids, for crying out loud—my brother wasn't even old enough to reach the stove. We ate a lot of ramen noodles, which are infamous for their high sodium content and complete absence of nutritional value. This went on for longer than anyone could have expected, and my brother and I both quietly ballooned in size. Along with physical girth, we both gained a host of new body image problems that would be a nuisance for years to come. Three major surgeries and nearly two decades later, my mom's health has greatly improved—but it took nearly that same amount of time for me and my brother to address the body image problems we accumulated during those dark days.

WHAT A CLICHÉ

As I pick through the emotional rubble from that *very* blue period in my family's life, I can find all the building blocks that eventually became the bedrock of my yoga practice.

I'm fully aware that my experience is the opposite of unique. For every maladjusted human being walking around on this planet, regardless of gender expression, there's a story just like mine. The details may vary, but the themes are basically the same: a cornucopia of self-imposed and society-endorsed body issues, with a barrage of unhealthy coping mechanisms sprinkled liberally on top.

I actually take a lot of comfort in the fact that this kind of sadness is such a common shared experience—ultimately, it's kind of the great unifier, isn't it? That's why I find it so strange that our shared alienation tends to be

---

7 I'm not joking about the musicals—from roughly 1996 to 1998, I made my little brother memorize most of the songs from *Annie*, *A Chorus Line*, all of the best songs from the straight-to-VHS collection of Olsen Twins detective comedies, and select musical performances from *The Little Rascals*. I have very clear memories of Gabriel playing the Molly to my Annie in our warbling renditions of "Maybe" and "You're Never Fully Dressed Without a Smile"— both of which are always classics, let's be real.

the first thing yoga teachers try to bury or hide while leading a class—they glorify life's sunshine and rainbows, but then completely fail to mention its dark, bittersweet moments. This baffles me because I think my yoga practice would be indescribably monotonous without the chaos of my daily life.

Because, make no mistake—I'm not naive.[8] I don't think the shitty parts of life are over for me just because I've cultivated a vigorous yoga practice. On the contrary, I think shitty things will continue to happen. But that's life. The fuckery never ends. Any attempts to control or anticipate the crests and valleys will only yield dissatisfaction and disappointment. Instead of trying to micromanage my emotional journey, I use yoga to pull up off the gas and help me see my life objectively and without judgement. It may not be foolproof, but it's the best tool I've found so far.

So maybe now you're thinking, "If yoga is so great, why isn't everyone all over it? Why is there such a narrow vision of yoga practitioners? Obviously it's not just wealthy white women who can benefit from the eight-limbed path, right?" I feel you, dude. I have thought these exact same thoughts. So enough about me and my "body issues"—for now, anyway. Let's get a better idea of what yoga actually is and how you can fit it into your own life.

---

8 Well, at least not *that* naive.

QUESTIONS ASKED BY (LITERALLY) EVERY BEGINNER YOGA STUDENT

WHAT IF MY BODY IS TOO WEAK TO PRACTICE ANY YOGA POSES AND I JUST FALL IN A HEAP ON THE FLOOR?

So, I hate to break it to you, but that will probably happen. More than once. It still happens to me all the time. Even after years of practicing, it's extremely common for yoga teachers to struggle just like any new practitioner. The difference is what happens when we face our weaknesses. For example, after falling into the aforementioned heap, did you continue to lie helplessly in a pool of your own sweat and tears, crying for someone to come pick you up and drag you out of yoga class? Or did you get back up and try the pose again? Everyone's body starts out at its own definition of weak—whether that weakness is physical, mental, or emotional. The most important part of practicing yoga is that even when our weaknesses cause us to fall, whether it's on or off the mat, are we able to strengthen ourselves in response? Are we able to gather our fears and learn from them?

I HAVE NO MOTIVATION TO EXERCISE AT ALL, LET ALONE PRACTICE YOGA. HOW CAN I MOTIVATE MYSELF?

Oh, motivation, you fickle little bitch. Motivation is a fairy-tale nymph— she dances in while we're feeling emotionally vulnerable in Dick's Sporting

Goods and encourages us to purchase expensive healthy living equipment thinking: "This time will be different." She buzzes around our heads while we're committing to expensive yoga class packages but conveniently pulls an abrupt dip out when we're silencing alarm clocks ten minutes before class.

I've become accustomed to motivation's inconsistent presence in my life, and I've accepted that it would be foolish to expect anything else. On days when I'm undermotivated, I can still remember how good the practice makes me feel and so I drag my ass to the mat. Once I get on my yoga mat, it doesn't matter if I'm motivated, because it would be too disappointing to put the mat away. That's my advice—just get on the mat. Don't expect to feel fully motivated every day; proceed full speed ahead without it. Soon, you'll realize that motivation is actually more like a car—really helpful if you have one, but you can find other ways to get around.

I'VE INJURED MY BODY AND I THINK IT WILL INHIBIT MY ABILITY TO PRACTICE YOGA. SHOULD I STILL GIVE IT A SHOT?

Early in my yoga practice, I dove headfirst into Urdhva Dhanurasana, otherwise known as Wheel Pose—it's a full spinal backbend requiring a remarkable amount of strength and conditioning in a variety of body parts, but particularly in the shoulders and wrists. I came of age in the *Bring It On* generation of competitive cheerleading and dancing, and this cheerleading mainstay became an early focus of my asana practice. Instead of considering my physical safety, I began practicing Wheel Pose without paying attention to my hand and wrist alignment. Over time, I noticed considerable pain in both of my wrist joints. Rather than rolling up my mat and putting my yoga practice on hold, I just adjusted my movements to accommodate my tender wrist joints—shorter holds in wrist-centric poses, or avoiding those poses entirely.

Simultaneously, I became obsessed with understanding my wrist joints—and the way I *should* have been placing my hands in order to avoid injury. I also began incorporating daily wrist stretches in my home practice (or, let's be real, semidaily—when it comes to adopting a consistent fitness regimen, this tiger has never changed her stripes). Over a period of months, I noticed my wrists becoming stronger and healthier. I'm still very careful with my wrists—I'm hesitant with arm balances and I constantly check my alignment when I'm flowing. However, my injury became the saving grace of my practice. It's how I learned to properly align myself in foundation yoga poses and it's allowed me to be much more mindful with my body.

That said, don't be reckless with your body. If you can take a class, get there early and describe your injury to your teacher so they can assist you with any necessary modifications. Don't do anything if it hurts. Don't push through pain.

But please do not see your injury as an impediment. I know, it's hard not to fall prey to our egos. And our egos tell us we have to be the most badass yoga student in class, performing every pose with the fluidity and ease of a young B. K. S. Iyengar. But even the great Iyengar struggled with injury—in fact, self-inflicted injuries from a harsh yoga practice led to his creation of the ubiquitous yoga lineage bearing his name. I could spend pages regaling you with stories of people who've healed life-altering injuries with a solid yoga practice, but it all boils down to a simple fact: Injuries happen. Change your perspective so that your injury isn't what holds you back, but what motivates you to greatness.

WHAT ARE THE SPIRITUAL BENEFITS?

I'm always weirded out when I'm asked this question, because the *entire experience* of practicing yoga is a spiritual one. (I go into the religious history of Ancient yoga on page 29.) Any yoga that "eliminates," "avoids," or "ignores" yoga's spiritual side is not *actually* yoga: It's a fitness routine in yoga clothing. Ultimately, the combined purpose of breath work, asana practice, and meditation is to lift us from our mental preoccupations and allow us to connect with our spirit or inner soul. This is spirituality that transcends any kind of religion, and being able to consistently tap into it provides unparalleled emotional and mental relief.

WILL YOGA HELP MY DEPRESSION?

I know that a consistent yoga practice can change lives—it's pulled people (myself included) out of hellishly dark mental and emotional circumstances. The focus, the breathing, the discipline. These are all really useful things when it comes to digging yourself out of emotional holes. But nothing is a silver bullet. There's no limit to the extent of suitable self-care for your own personal life hurricane. If you're really struggling, talk to a professionally trained therapist, psychiatrist, or counselor to help you sort through emotional damage and trauma. Do that AND do yoga. Your practice will continue to buoy you *while your life continues to unfold*. It doesn't make the bad stuff go away, but it can help you deal with it.

CAN I DO YOGA IF I'M "OLD"?

Yoga has absolutely no age limits. Practitioners of all ages are more than welcome. Ideally, a person would begin practicing yoga immediately after birth and continue to grow their practice over the course of their entire life. No matter when you come to your mat, you can build a practice that works for you and your body. Start with this book or start with a class. If you're taking a class for the first time, go early to talk with the teacher. Be up front but unapologetic and unconcerned about any perceived physical limitations and then take it from there.

I'M IN A WHEELCHAIR AND I WANT TO PRACTICE YOGA. WHERE DO I START?

Certain parts of this book may read like The Ableist's Guide to Yoga. I call out specific body parts all the time, and there are very few modifications offered for those with difficulty standing. That being said, YOU CAN STILL DO YOGA. Believe me—just because you're sitting down doesn't mean you can't adapt all these poses to your bodily circumstance. If you're able to stand, but you need additional support to keep yourself upright while practicing standing postures, practicing yoga poses next to a wall or with a sturdy chair can work wonders and make a myriad of yoga poses accessible. Throughout yoga practice, you can press your hand/foot/spine into a wall for additional support, or use a chair or couch for the exact same purpose. If you're in a wheelchair or unable to stand, make upper-body yoga your focus. If you can do the arm actions of a given pose but not the leg actions (or vice versa), that's perfectly fine. Just make it work for you, even if your body doesn't look anything like the pictures. Also, simply closing your eyes and shutting off a visual connection to the outside world can work wonders in altering perspective. Your yoga journey is absolutely equal to anyone else's, even if your body has a different physical presentation. If you're looking for specific guidance, I'd recommend grabbing a copy of Edeltraud Rohnfeld's *Chair Yoga: Seated Exercises for Health and Wellbeing*.

I REALLY WANT TO LOSE WEIGHT—WILL YOGA WORK FOR ME?

Short answer? Yes, it will definitely work for you. Long answer? Yoga is a lot of things, but it's not a weight loss plan. The purpose is not and will never be to control your body weight. It's definitely likely that the combined effect of a vigorous yoga practice and a healthy diet will result in changes in body composition. But the best overall results of a yoga practice come when the practitioner does not focus on one specific reason for coming to the mat. If you devote yourself to a yoga practice solely for the purposes of seeing within yourself, living the eight-limbed path (page 35), and communing with the world around you, your body will feel all the positive results you've ever wanted to experience.

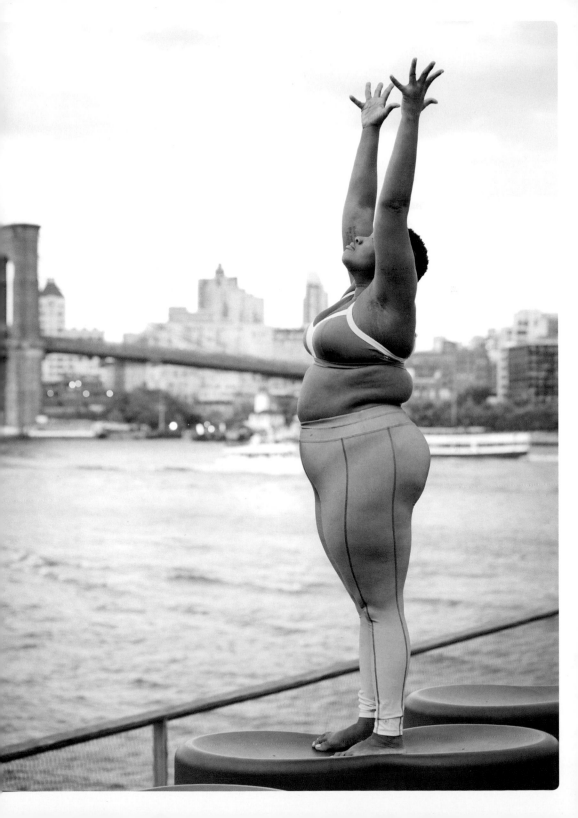

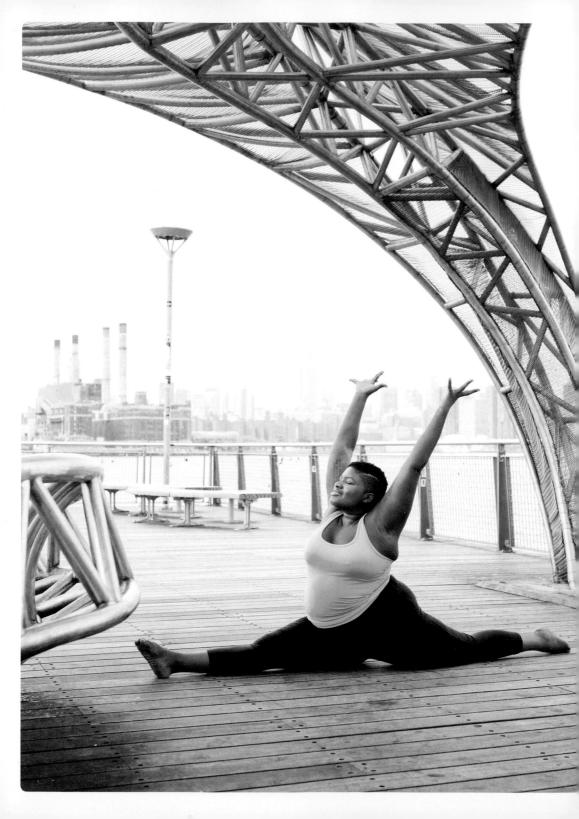

PART 2

What the Hell Is This?

THE HISTORY OF MODERN YOGA, IN A NUTSHELL

Yoga means "to yolk"—it's an ancient life practice that's all about the union and discipline of a person's spirit, body, and mind. The physical practice makes our bodies strong and bendy, as well as providing respiratory, circulatory, digestive, and hormonal relief. Simultaneously, the breathing and meditation practices allow us to manifest a deeper emotional and spiritual connection to the world around us.

Yoga is a beautiful practice, but it's frequently misunderstood and often misinterpreted. If polled at random, a diverse group of yoga practitioners would likely offer a wide array of conflicting answers about both the origin and nature of yoga. Some practitioners would probably say it's simply a physical fitness exercise, while others might swear it's a devotional spiritual practice. Both of these ideological camps can be correct. But let me make a few distinctions right off the bat.

For one thing, even though they are obviously related, there is a very clear difference between the ancient practice of yoga, which is heavy with religious and cultural context, and the largely secular modern practice of yoga, which is characterized more by fitness (and consumerism) than religion. There isn't one of these yogic "denominations" that's better than the other. There isn't one that's wrong or bad. These yogic schools are *not*, however, interchangeable.

WHAT ARE THE MAJOR DIFFERENCES BETWEEN ANCIENT YOGA AND MODERN YOGA?

	ANCIENT YOGA	MODERN YOGA
How old is it?	Ancient yoga is several thousand years old, and it originated in India. Ancient practitioners were known for separating themselves from the rest of society and leading nomadic lives fully dedicated to understanding the union of their mind, body, and spirit.	Modern yoga began to surface around the turn of the twentieth century, a time when a small number of Eastern yoga gurus traveled to Europe and the Americas spreading various styles of both athletic and nonathletic yoga.
Is this stuff religious?	Yes, yoga was, and still is, heavily woven into the social and cultural structure of India. In the past, it was a way for a practitioner to ascend India's caste system and improve the options allowed to them in their daily life and in the afterlife. You can find specific references to yoga within multiple religious faiths of Eastern origin, including Hinduism, Buddhism, and Jainism.	No, Modern yoga is not specifically religious. Practitioners can be found across the entire spectrum of religious belief, from the most devout Catholics to the most skeptical atheists. Modern yoga allows practitioners to retain their unique cultural identities while still pursuing a life on the yogic path.
Is it unisex?	Ancient yoga was notoriously patriarchal, and women were not allowed to practice until the early twentieth century.	Modern yoga is women-centric, with the largest percentage of practitioners identifying with traditional cisgender female pronouns.

WHAT ARE THE MAJOR DIFFERENCES BETWEEN ANCIENT YOGA AND MODERN YOGA?

	ANCIENT YOGA	MODERN YOGA
How many styles are there?	The ancient yogis outlined four specific paths of self-discernment (i.e., four paths to understanding your existence on Earth): **jnana marga** (a path of knowledge), **karma marga** (a path of selfless service), **bhakti marga** (a path of love and devotion), and **yoga marga** (a path of bringing the mind's action under control). All paths lead to a state of bliss. Asana (poses) are not considered to be essential; more emphasis is placed upon meditation and breathing, as well as internal and external cleanliness.	Too many to name here (see page 42), although practice of asana is frequently considered to be essential. Modern yoga styles typically draw influences from the ancient paths of spiritual self-discernment, but they are also characterized by the personal philosophies of their respective gurus/creators. Many are heavily influenced by Western fitness culture.
How is it taught?	Ancient yoga wasn't taught in classes—it was a one-on-one exchange between an experienced and influential guru and his student.	Modern yoga is typically a group learning experience, and large group classes have become the norm across the West.
Is it materialistic?	No. Most practitioners were encouraged to live an ascetic life, free of ties to financial wealth and greed.	Yes. The culture surrounding Modern yoga lineages places a heavy emphasis on the acquisition of yoga-related goods and services.

As a practitioner of Modern hatha yoga, I consider two major Ancient yogic texts to form the bedrock of my yoga practice: Swatmarama's *Hatha Yoga Pradipika* (written in the fifteenth century) and Sage Patanjali's *The Yoga Sutras of Patanjali* (from around 400 CE).

The Yoga Sutras outlines a path for becoming one with the divine. In it, Patanjali lays out an eight-limbed path of yoga, a step-by-step approach to freedom from all suffering. *Pradipika*, on the other hand, was the first book to ever *really* talk about yoga asana. Swatmarama outlined fewer than twenty poses that were meant to help with meditation, digestion, and harnessing centralized energy. For hundreds of years, yoga students and gurus studied and meditated on these texts, handing down the ancient wisdom from person to person.

In the 1920s, an influential yoga guru named Tirumalai Krishnamacharya began teaching asana yoga classes in the gymnasiums of Mysore, India. Krishnamacharya's practice was a flow of athletic asana that we now call vinyasa yoga. His classes were predominantly attended by energetic young boys whose parents were looking for a way to quiet their overactive minds and bodies. In essence, Krishnamacharya's yoga classes served as Depression-era Ritalin. His unique blend of traditional Hatha Yoga Pradipika asana mixed with European gymnastics and calisthenics became popular in India and spread to the West. Because of his influence over such a large number of students across both the East and West, Krishnamacharya is widely considered to be the father of Modern yoga.

Several of Krishnamacharya's students went on to be prolific yoga gurus in their own rights. One of his students, Sri K. Pattabhi Jois, went on to found the wildly popular discipline of Ashtanga yoga, a highly athletic yogic path. B. K. S. Iyengar, who was both student *and* brother-in-law of Krishnamacharya, created an eponymous style of yoga that places a heavy emphasis on proper alignment of the body and encourages the use of props.[9] Both of these great teachers brought their particular styles to the US,

---

9 Prior to Mr. Iyengar, yoga props basically didn't exist—he created them in a very DIY fashion to ease injuries he'd sustained through years of Krishnamacharya's sometimes brutal yoga sequencing.

and Ashtanga and Iyengar yoga have since become some of the most ubiquitous styles of yoga in the West. A plethora of Modern yoga styles proudly claim Iyengarian and Ashtangan techniques as the basis of their practice, including Jivamukti, Anusara, and Forrest yoga.

However, it's unlikely that Modern yoga would exist in its current form without one of Krishnamacharya's most unlikely students, Indra Devi. Devi was a Russian-born actress and socialite, and in the 1930s her studentship was foisted upon Krishnamacharya. Despite the fact that yoga was rarely taught to non-Indians and essentially never taught to women, the great yoga guru's patrons, the royal family of Mysore, India, insisted he take her on. Devi eventually became one of Krishnamacharya's most prized pupils, and she traveled the world spreading her guru's brand of yoga. By the 1950s, Devi had brought yoga to Los Angeles, the epicenter of American glamour and materialism, and she famously taught Hollywood stars like Gloria Swanson and Greta Garbo. But for the most part, yoga remained on the fringes of Western culture until Hollywood found it again in the late 1990s, with pop culture icons like Madonna, Willem Dafoe, Jennifer Aniston, and Gwyneth Paltrow bowing at the proverbial knee of Ashtanga's Sri K. Pattabhi Jois, as well as other prominent Modern yoga gurus, such as Sharon Gannon and David Life, founders of Jivamukti Yoga.

Over the course of the twentieth century and into the twenty-first century, Modern yoga gurus have established niche communities of practitioners all over the world. There are almost as many styles of Modern yoga as there are practitioners on this planet (see page 42). Many are a hybrid of traditional yoga asana and philosophy and other styles of movement, such as ballet, capoeira, tai chi, aerial arts, hip-hop, and modern dance,

guru is a Sanskrit word meaning "teacher, guide, expert, or master." A guru is a reverential figure who serves as a spiritual guide for the student.

yogi refers to a practitioner of yoga who is fully devoted to the eight-limbed path.

among others. But Modern yoga is distinguished from Ancient yoga by its cultural context, its absence of direct religious influence, and its gender specifications. Modern yoga also tends to place a much more substantial emphasis on the physical benefits of a regular asana practice, as opposed to the cumulative benefits of the eight-limbed path.

More complicated is the fact that Modern yoga bears the unmistakable influence of stereotypical Western values such as a focus on physical beauty and materialism. These values don't seem to be shared by Ancient yoga, as it enjoys a more obviously ascetic and spiritual value systems. However, Modern yoga has evolved into a beautiful mélange of varied perspectives and techniques, with a diverse cornucopia of practitioners. It's truly a salute to the amazing diversity of our global melting pot.

WHAT THE FUCK IS THE EIGHT-LIMBED PATH?

One of the downsides of Modern yoga is that it tends to place primary focus on the physical yoga asana practice, which can evolve into a general disregard for the importance of yoga's nonphysical aspects. There are a ton of people who practice yoga asana on a regular basis, but who are clueless about the eight-limbed path. And even though asana is amazing (so amazing that multiple sections of this book are devoted to it), it's not really the *most* important part overall. It's an awesome limb, but it's legit only one out of eight. Frankly, up until Krishnamacharya got involved, asana was considered a fairly unimportant part of the yogic path.[10]

Here's the thing—even if you don't read any other books about yoga, get a copy of *The Yoga Sutras of Patanjali* and devour it immediately. Around 400 CE, an ancient yoga sage named Patanjali made a number of profound observations about the nature of humanity and society at large.[11] His observations were then collected into what's known as *The Yoga Sutras,* and those same observations have remained relevant

---

10 If you skipped the section about yoga history, skip back to page 29, playa.

11 Whether or not Patanjali was a single person is up for debate—many scholars believe the "sage Patanjali" is really just a title given to a number of people who collectively accumulated the sutras over a long period of time.

characterizations of humanity up until and including the present day. Collectively, the sutras outline the eight-limbed path of yoga, also known as Ashtanga yoga. Patanjali basically thought that by following the eight-limbed path, yoga practitioners would be freed from the suffering of our external world. All limbs of the path are meant to create an integrated web of internal discernment to guide our actions on a daily basis. It breaks down like this:

1. YAMAS (RESTRAINTS)

Yamas remind us of our responsibilities to others. They are divided into five "principles."

- **Ahimsa (nonviolence):** Be full of compassion, introspection, and self-restraint when approaching fellow beings and your own body.

- **Satya (truthfulness):** Don't lie. Always tell the truth and live in truth, even when it hurts. Always speak directly and act with intention.

- **Asteya (freedom from covetousness):** Don't yearn for other people's shit. Be cool with who you are and don't make yourself into the image of someone else.

- **Brahmacharya (chastity):** Don't throw your sexuality to the wind. Discipline your sexual life so that you only seek contentment and moral strength from within *yourself*, instead of from *other people*.

- **Aparigraha (freedom from desire):** Don't be a greedy asshole. Don't associate possessions with happiness or self-worth.

2. NIYAMAS (DISCIPLINE)

Niyamas remind us of our responsibilities to ourselves. Like the yamas, there are five "principles."

- **Saucha (cleanliness):** Keep your body clean—physically, mentally, AND emotionally.

- **Santosa (contentment):** Be happy and content in the present moment. Do not long for the past or obsess over the future. Just be right here, right now.

- **Tapas (austerity):** Build heat within yourself, via meditation or asana, in order to yield self-discipline and the ultimate sense of honesty.

- **Svadhyaya (study of the self):** Look within yourself for the answers to life's questions. By studying the self, we can be more mindful and conscious of the role we play in the universe at large.

- **Ishvara Pranidhana (devotion to god):** Devote yourself fully to the (religion-free) divinity ever present in the universe and all beings therein.

3. ASANA (AKA THE YOGA POSES THAT EVERYONE, THEIR MOTHER, AND THEIR MOTHER'S MOTHER HAVE BECOME OBSESSED WITH LEARNING)

The purpose of asana is to generate energy within the inner body to strengthen and purify the self as a whole. At the end of the day, a "perfect" yoga pose is performed when the practitioner is able to breathe with ease while in a state of action, and the pose itself effectively becomes effortless. There will still be shaking, trembling, and other bodily fluctuations, but the goal for the practitioner is to accept that fluctuations are an unavoidable aspect of their practice—and their life.

4. PRANAYAMA (BREATH WORK)

What's often trivialized as "just breathing" is actually a pretty epic action. *Prana* means "vital energy" and *ayama* means "stretch, expansion, and extension"—in essence, you're stretching vital energy through your body. Does that sound trivial to you? Regular pranayama practice is crucial not just in an asana or meditation practice, but in every other part of life—when we take even one minute to breathe mindfully and thoughtfully, it's possible to completely shift our perspectives.

5. PRATYAHARA (DETACHMENT FROM THE EXTERNAL)

Pratyahara is a hard one for us Westerners. We have a nearly devotional attachment to the external—our looks, our possessions, our total immersion in the digital world. By detaching, practitioners are able to pull away from all that mindless chatter and, in doing so, reject the fears, concerns, and absorptions that consume our daily lives. Our minds become passive and we clear away the clutter of our senses.

6. DHARANA (CONCENTRATION)

By this point in the path, the practitioner has come to understand that divinity originates within. In order to access this ever-present divinity, it's necessary for the practitioner to find a point of focus in order to direct their mind and body into a meditative state. Imagine a pirouetting ballet dancer, spinning on a point and using a singular point of focus as a mark to maintain focus. In that same way, as one walks along the eight-limbed path of yoga, it is helpful to establish an internal point of focus, such as closing the eyes during dhyana (meditation) and establishing a gaze at an invisible "third eye" located between the two physical eyes.

7. DHYANA (MEDITATION)

At its core, meditation is merely an honest experience of quiet and peace. By remaining quiet, we release attachment and become untethered to both the pleasures and woes of life. In meditation, there is no sadness or happiness—only acceptance. When we make a habit of accepting the parts of life that upset us, we are able to renounce the feelings of unhappiness or displeasure that regularly manifest in our external lives.

8. SAMADHI (TOTAL ABSORPTION)

Samadhi is the state of absolute balance of the mind, body, and spirit, and it is the ultimate goal of the eight-limbed path. Once the practitioner has fully absorbed the other seven limbs, they release the immature and ego-driven desires of their small mind and come into a complete union with the ever-present (and religion-free) divinity of all creations. This isn't a quick journey, and the experience of samadhi is directly linked to the eight-limbed path's application to a practitioner's unique and individual lifestyle. But once a practitioner arrives at the gates of samadhi, there is nothing else to strive for and nothing else to "need."

My own eight-limbed path has slowly revealed itself—and it still morphs and changes with every passing day. Like that of most Modern yoga practitioners, my eight-limbed path began with an insatiable obsession with asana. However, as I've begun incorporating the other limbs into my life, particularly dhyana (meditation) and the niyama of santosa (contentment), my incorrigible narcissism has evolved from an Achilles heel to a lens for understanding the ways in which I approach the world.

Ideally, once you assume your own unique walk down the eight-limbed path, it should become a guiding force of your life—both on and off the yoga mat. A true practitioner walks the eight-limbed path until their final breath.

WHICH YOGA PRACTICE SHOULD I CHOOSE?

There are (basically) a million different styles of Modern yoga asana practices. Modern yoga lineages are highly influenced by or directly descended from Hatha yoga, with an emphasis on physical asana practice over other limbs of the eight-limbed paths. Some lineages are highly athletic, some are highly restorative; some emphasize props, some emphasize alignment. Some practitioners follow one specific yoga lineage and feel a very strong connection with the teachings of a few specific people. Latching on to a specific yoga lineage, with its individual set of rituals, chants, alignment techniques, and lifestyle goals, can give practitioners a tangible sense of heritage and community, but no single asana path is the *only* yogic path. I believe that there's value in incorporating a wide variety of asana styles into your practice. Each style of yoga offers different physical, emotional, and spiritual benefits, and blending several styles of yoga together gives you a practice that can move seamlessly with the ups and downs of your daily life.

In the end, you're looking for balance. That means stepping out of your comfort zone and trying styles of yoga that don't immediately appeal to you. Sometimes, doing shit you don't want to do can yield the best results.

In my humble opinion, the best and most fulfilling yoga asana practices incorporate an equal balance of both yin- and yang-style poses. Yang-style yoga flows are very common in Modern yoga—they place primary focus upon fast-paced, vigorous, and dynamic postural movements that build internal heat and strengthen muscular composition. Yin-style yoga sequencing, which highlights elements of Chinese Taoist philosophy, places a greater emphasis on joint and ligament composition by using slow, long postural holds to stretch and strengthen connective tissue. By placing equal emphasis on both yin- and yang-style asana, practitioners can create a sense of internal harmony throughout their asana practices and beyond.

I've outlined a few of the more prominent Modern yoga lineages on the following pages. You may notice that I essentially say that all of these styles of yoga are hard. That's because . . . yoga asana is difficult. Honestly, it's *meant* to be difficult. If the asana wasn't challenging, we would miss the point of practicing yoga. Just because something is hard doesn't mean it's bad. Go to class with an open mind and you will reap all the benefits. Mix and match classes, studios, and teachers—a diverse yoga education is the key to a balanced practice.

What follows is the quick-and-dirty edition. I encourage you to read more. Even the most experienced yoga teachers are always reading, taking classes, and finding new opportunities to learn from their own teachers and students. There are several books that I consider standard fare if you're interested in taking your yoga practice to the next level.

• *Light on Yoga* and *Yoga: The Path to Holistic Health*, both by B. K. S. Iyengar

• *Yoga Anatomy, 2nd Edition*, by Leslie Kaminoff & Amy Matthews

• *The Bhagavad Gita*, translated by Stephen Mitchell

• *The Yoga Sutras of Patanjali*, translated by Sri Swami Satchidananda

• *Yoga: The Spirit and Practice of Moving into Stillness*, by Erich Schiffmann

Once you dive into these other texts, your increased knowledge can't help but lead to a stronger overall practice.

WHAT YOGA STYLES SHOULD I BLEND TOGETHER
FOR THE PERFECT PRACTICE?

STYLE	WHAT IS IT?	WHO MIGHT ENJOY IT?	WILL IT KICK MY ASS?
Anusara	An alignment-oriented yoga and philosophical practice focused on opening up parts of your body in order to become more graceful, energetic, and free.	Anyone seeking an alignment-oriented full-body experience, along with a spiritual practice guided by the principles of tantrism.	Yes, but you will learn a lot about alignment, and you'll encounter a myriad of "Anusara-specific" ways to open your heart.
Ashtanga Vinyasa	A highly athletic practice that combines gymnastic-like moves, deep breath work, long holds, and repetitive transitions.	Anyone who likes to sweat, have their ass kicked, and learn powerful life lessons along the way.	Yes, but if you're looking for visible physical results in an asana practice, there's hardly a better practice. Plus, the practice demands a sense of self-discipline that will inevitably cross over to the rest of your life.
Bikram	A specific sequence of 26 asana performed in a room heated to about 105 degrees.	Literally anyone—the Bikram sequence is designed to be approachable by a wide range of people, though the combination of heat and very long pose holds can be intimidating to new practitioners.	Yes, but the extreme heat allows your body to be softer and more flexible than it would be in a typical non-hot class. Plus, sweating is really good for your body's overall condition.

WHAT YOGA STYLES SHOULD I BLEND TOGETHER FOR THE PERFECT PRACTICE?

STYLE	WHAT IS IT?	WHO MIGHT ENJOY IT?	WILL IT KICK MY ASS?
Forrest	Influenced by Ashtanga, Iyengar, Sivananda yoga style, and traditional Native American medicine work, Forrest yoga utilizes long holds, intensive core work, and a strong standing asana series to unlock buried physical and emotional trauma.	Anyone with a vested interest in using their yoga as a tool to unlock buried trauma and emotional distress.	YES. The core work alone means that this style of yoga is definitely an ass-kicker. But it works on your body like a deep tissue massage—the longer you stay in the poses and the more you turn up the internal heat, the looser both your body and spirit become, and the more supple you become overall.
Iyengar	Developed by B. K. S. Iyengar after he sustained a yoga-related injury, this practice puts heavy emphasis on alignment, prop modification, and breath work.	Anyone with a strong interest in anatomy or who wants to learn the keys to resolving long-term physical distress.	Don't let the props fool you into thinking Iyengar meant for his yoga to be easy—because of its alignment centricity and long holds, this style of yoga can definitely kick your ass.

WHAT YOGA STYLES SHOULD I BLEND TOGETHER FOR THE PERFECT PRACTICE?

STYLE	WHAT IS IT?	WHO MIGHT ENJOY IT?	WILL IT KICK MY ASS?
Jivamukti	A dynamic vinyasa-style practice that places equal emphasis on asana, scripture, devotion, music, and meditation. There is a heavy emphasis on ahimsa (page 36), the yama of nonviolence, and this is characterized by adherence to a vegan lifestyle, as well as animal rights and environmental activism.	Anyone seeking a strong and dynamic asana practice that also offers a tightly woven community of environmentally and socially conscious fellow practitioners.	While the physical practice can be quite demanding, Jivamukti's true complexities come in embodying the lifestyle as a whole.
Kundalini	A deeply spiritual practice with an emphasis on unlocking and cherishing a student's kundalini energy, envisioned as a coiled snake resting at the base of the spine, and opening the seven bodily chakras to create a communion with the universe.	While the physical practice can be arduous, the spiritual work of Kundalini yoga tends to draw students who seek a greater connection to their internal spiritual composition and the universe around them.	Because of its heavy emphasis on breath work, meditation, energy work, and focus, Kundalini yoga has a tendency to be much more difficult than anticipated.

WHAT YOGA STYLES SHOULD I BLEND TOGETHER FOR THE PERFECT PRACTICE?

STYLE	WHAT IS IT?	WHO MIGHT ENJOY IT?	WILL IT KICK MY ASS?
Vinyasa	A dance-like, flow-style practice that uses the linking of breath and movement to create sequences that highlight the transient nature of the human form. There are many variations, including Power and Baptiste.	Anyone who wants to unlock their inner modern dancer while learning about their true self.	Yoga-style dancing paired with deep breathing? Yes, this style can definitely take the wind out of your sails. But classes are typically lighthearted, and many include secular music.
Yin/ Restorative	A slower-paced practice with emphasis on meditative, long holds—poses are usually held for about five minutes each. Props and modifications are commonly utilized to increase bodily circulation and flexibility.	Anyone who needs to take a moment, breathe, and just chill. Even when the poses are intense, they will absolutely require that you *chill*.	Though it is more slow-paced than other Modern yoga styles, yin yoga shouldn't be written off as easy—because the pose holds are so long, the practice can ultimately turn out to be more physically and emotionally demanding than most styles.

A WORD ON IDENTITY AND APPROPRIATION

As devoted to our yoga practice as we Westerners may be, we need to remain conscious of the offense that can come when we appropriate aspects of South Asian culture that are not solely connected to the yoga world. There are a million ways this can happen, and no Western yoga practitioners should consider themselves exempt from Eastern yoga cultural appropriation, even if it is accidental. One of my favorite examples is the now-quintessential image of a Western white woman donning an Indian bindi and sari for a yoga ritual within her chosen yoga lineage. While this may seem an innocuous gesture, and perhaps even a respectful display of admiration, it could simultaneously be viewed by a South Asian person as an intentional theft and mockery of their cultural identity.

When building your own Modern yoga practice, regardless of lineage, remember to remain discerning about the aspects of Ancient yoga and South Asian culture that you choose to claim for your own. For example, the teachings of sages like Patanjali and Swatmarama can be adapted for any lifestyle, regardless of religious, cultural, or social demographics. Those teachings, however, should be interpreted within the unique sociocultural identity and lifestyle of the practitioner. My hope is that a new generation of discerning secular practitioners will make the offensive appropriation of South Asian culture a distant memory.

WHAT SHOULD I BUY?

I've often joked that when someone asks, "How do I start practicing yoga?" what they're really asking is, "What should I *buy* in order to start practicing yoga?"

Now, I can't tell a lie—I take full ownership of my twenty-first-century yoga yuppie-dom. I mean, I subscribe to *Yoga Journal*. I own more yoga mats and yoga tools than one individual could ever reasonably need. I have two full dresser drawers full of only yoga leggings. However, these *things* have nothing to do with my practice. I don't need two dresser drawers of yoga leggings. I don't even need a yoga mat in order to practice. And while I do love staying up to date on what's going on in the yoga world, the information in *Yoga Journal* isn't the backbone of my practice. Ultimately, the focus of a yoga practice should be adherence to the eight-limbed path in one's daily life.

But let's be real, shall we? Yoga mats are cool, and buying stuff can be really fucking fun. Especially if you're really digging into a yoga practice, and you're the type that likes to accessorize. And honestly, I think that yoga is even more fun when you accessorize. If you want to be smart about your yoga supplies, there are a few things you need to know.

NOT ALL YOGA MATS ARE CREATED EQUAL

It should be stated that mats are absolutely NOT a requirement for practicing yoga. They do, however, make things A LOT easier. I would say they make practicing asana both easier and better on virtually every kind of surface, from carpet to gravel to hardwood to linoleum.

Not all yoga mats are created equal. Unfortunately, the best mats are expensive, but that doesn't necessarily mean cheapo mats are all bad. When I started practicing yoga, I was just using my dad's old Pilates mat. It was the kind of mat that comes in one of those yoga starter kits you might find on a holiday endcap at Target or Walmart. It was relatively thin (3mm), of standard length and width (68" x 24"), and very, *very* slippery. I would drape a towel over it to absorb the intense sweatstorm dripping from every inch of my body. I slipped around a little, but things were steady enough for me and my meager-ass budget. Honestly, I simply couldn't afford to spend extra money on a yoga mat.

That was my yoga mat setup for about two years. Eventually, I saved my pennies and invested in a high-end mat about five millimeters thick, and a little longer than your average yoga mat. I appreciated the extra few inches of mat space because, as a curvy person, I like to have a little extra space, ya dig? The mat is dual-sided—one side is perfect for practicing in non-hot classes, and the other side is perfect for hot classes, as it actually gets "grippier" as your body gets sweatier!

For new students, I recommend buying a cheapo mat and throwing a towel over it. You will be fine. I promise. And when your practice deepens and you want to invest in a really amazing mat that will take your asana practice to another level, well then treat yo' self to a really fucking nice mat. Something that will be extremely grippy, cushy, and very spacious. Buy yourself a mat that will make you *really* excited to practice yoga. Sometimes the very simple gesture of buying yourself a really nice yoga mat can be the key to a yoga practice really getting off the ground.

PROP THAT ASS UP

I think yoga props are pretty amazing. By using blocks, straps, bolsters, pillows, blankets, wedges, benches, and a wide array of other objects to support your body, you can make your yoga asana and meditation practices deeper and more satisfying. And that goes for EVERY human body, not just those with sensitive knees, replaced hip joints, spinal injuries, or any other combination of bodily quirks. Even the most "physically fit" person, someone with a liquid spine and rubber muscles, would find great benefit from using yoga props in their practice.

I wasn't introduced to the magic of yoga props until pretty deep in my practice. My foundational yoga knowledge was established in Bikram studios, and Bikram yoga doesn't utilize yoga props at all. When I transitioned to practicing yoga at home, I couldn't really afford to buy any new yoga stuff and I didn't think the props could make a difference. However, as time went on, I discovered how helpful it could be to have the occasional yoga block under my hand in Extended Triangle Pose (page 87) or a strap when attempting Extended Hand to Big Toe Pose (page 92).

At the time, I grabbed random household objects to fill in the gap: my very first yoga strap was a raggedy nylon dog leash, and my first yoga blocks were stacked hardcover copies of *The Joy of Cooking* and *Harry Potter and the Deathly Hallows*. Eventually, I got a little classier and upgraded my yoga strap to an old chiffon-ish burgundy scarf and a homemade crocheted strap made by mother. My yoga block collection grew to include a heavily duct-taped *Star Wars* VHS box set as well as a couple of cell phone boxes bound together with packing tape. I used blankets covered in dog hair to cushion my sitting bones in Seated Forward Bend (page 125), and my early bolsters were nothing more than bed pillows.

No matter which avenue you choose, DIY/upcycled or Branded Gear, don't be afraid to prop that shit up. I would recommend that *every* yoga student, regardless of style, always have a few of the following items on hand.

ITEM	HOW MANY?	WHY?	OKAY, BUT DO I HAVE TO BUY IT?
Yoga blocks	2 to 4	Because your arms and legs won't magically grow longer, and yoga blocks can offer a boost.	Nah. Although I definitely recommend actual yoga blocks because of their design strengths, you can easily substitute a stack of books or a cleverly MacGuyvered tower of boxes to get the job done.
Yoga strap	1 to 2	Because you shouldn't have to mentally torture yourself in order to reach one of your limbs. Plus, straps can be used to keep your muscles engaged in poses like Dolphin Pose (page 99).	An old necktie, a discarded polyester scarf, a badly worn dog leash—these are all yoga straps in disguise.
Blanket	1 to 2	Because it can be nice to cushion your joints, like in Low Lunge Pose (page 106), or support your lower back, like in Seated Forward Bend (page 125). Also, you might get chilly in Corpse Pose (page 130).	Just go grab your comforter. It's not that serious, I promise. I have never purchased a yoga blanket, and I'm not sad about it.
Bolster	1 to 2	Because it can make your back feel amazing, and it can instantly make a lot of asana feel very restorative.	I mean, pillows are dope, but they are a little too squishy to make great long-term bolsters. You want your bolster to be a little stiff and rigid so it provides good resistance in restorative shapes. Frankly, the best bolsters… are bolsters.

YOGA CLOTHES—TO EACH THEIR OWN

In my opinion, comfort is the most important thing to consider when selecting yoga clothes. For me, that means wearing skintight, breathable clothing that allows me to easily manipulate my flesh and see what my body is doing. For you, that might mean wearing loose, soft clothing that makes you feel cozy. To each their own. Just remember to pick clothes based upon what makes YOU feel good, not what you think will make other people feel comfortable. It should be said that baggier clothing can become problematic when practicing inverted asana—it's not exactly fun when a baggy T-shirt covers your eyes during Supported Headstand (page 101).

When I practice in studios, my typical yoga outfit is either long, tight leggings or very short booty shorts paired with a sports bra. As long as you abide by the dress code of your local studio, wear whatever the fuck makes you feel good.

When I practice at home, I like to wear as few clothes as possible. Honestly, I've always appreciated opportunities to be in the buff or seminude, and practicing yoga is the perfect opportunity to enjoy some time in your birthday suit. When you practice while wearing minimal or no clothes, you lose the distraction of fashion and instead find some peace with your bodily composition. You can look at every freckle, curve, bruise, and stretch mark without disdain. I am convinced that a nude or seminude yoga practice is one of the unspoken keys to a better relationship with the body as a whole.

QUESTIONS ASKED BY (LITERALLY) EVERY BEGINNER YOGA STUDENT

I BIT THE BULLET AND I'M GOING TO MY FIRST YOGA CLASS. I'M NERVOUS. WHAT CAN I EXPECT?

Before you show up to the yoga studio, make sure you've got a few essentials on deck: mat, water bottle, and (if you're a "sweaty" person like me) a hand towel. If you're going to a hot yoga class, especially a Bikram class, pack a full-length towel to drape across your mat as a way to soak up body sweat or wipe sweat off your body.

Wear breathable and comfortable clothing. (I talk about the best yoga clothes on the previous page.) Leave your shoes outside the studio, and I wouldn't recommend wearing socks.

Keep your cell phone in your car, the studio lobby—frankly, anywhere but in the actual yoga room. Hearing a cell phone ring during yoga class is very distracting, and leaving your phone at the door is a sign of respect to your fellow practitioners.

When you enter the yoga studio, even if there isn't a lobby, there will always be someone present to check students in and accept class payment. This person may be the teacher, a receptionist, or maybe a work-study student. During the check-in process, the teacher may ask you questions about your yoga history—whether or not you've practiced before, if you have any injuries of note, etc. Don't feel pressured to give more information than makes you comfortable, but this is the time to tell your teacher about anything that may be causing you anxiety—your lack of experience, a rusty knee joint, or that you don't like for people to touch you . . . at all.[12]

When you walk into the yoga room, roll out your mat and, if available, get yourself set up with a few yoga props. If you have major issues with balance, it wouldn't hurt to set your mat up near a wall so you can use it to help keep you steady. Props are not a sign of weakness—they are a way to strengthen your practice. Don't be shy or embarrassed about setting yourself up with a couple of blocks, a bolster, a blanket, and a strap. (I talk more about props on page 49.)

Before the class begins, I like to just breathe quietly in Corpse Pose (page 130) or cross-legged on my mat. Some people like to "warm up" before the class gets going, but I've never found this to be necessary. The most important warm-up you can give yourself is to establish a clear and firm connection with your ujjayi breath (page 65). It will help relax and center you for what's to come.

The class itself may knock your socks off—and that's perfectly fine. You may experience a lot of sensations and emotions that are physically debilitating—and that's also fine. Feel comfortable dropping down to your knees if Downward-Facing Dog (page 80) becomes too intense, or pulling back into Child's Pose (page 124) if you can't catch your breath. The most important thing is that you find ways to maintain your even, steady breath. If you're having difficulty keeping up with the class pace, don't berate yourself. Just take a few breaths to watch the instructor. Sometimes it takes us a while to catch the rhythm of a yoga flow (ESPECIALLY if you're a brand-new practitioner) and ain't no shame in watching more than physically moving.

---

12 *Information like this can sometimes lead to your teacher giving you a lot of attention throughout the class. Personally, I hate receiving excess attention while practicing yoga, so I will always be the last person to offer information about my body and yoga history. But if it makes you feel more comfortable, let 'em know what's going on with your body.*

By the way, don't skip out on the final Corpse Pose (page 130) that ends the class. Sealing in your practice with a rest is a crucial part of the asana experience.

THERE ARE VERY FEW YOGA STUDIOS AROUND ME, AND NONE OF THEM KNOW HOW TO WORK WITH A BIGGER-BODIED STUDENT. WHAT SHOULD I DO?

As much as I'd like to say "just give every studio a chance," I can't. I know what it's like to enter a studio that is nowhere near body positive—studios that prefer Western fitness values over yogic philosophy. It can be extremely disheartening and discouraging, and with class drop-in rates averaging around twenty dollars a pop, you shouldn't waste your money on a lackluster experience. I would recommend retreating to the most body-positive studio of all time: your home. I know it can seem intimidating to begin a home practice, especially if you've had difficulty maintaining a fitness regimen in the past. Trust me, I've been there. I can't count the number of unsuccessful attempts I've made at sticking to Weight Watchers, Couch to 5K, and a host of other fitness lifestyle programs. However, when you make a commitment to yourself that doesn't have anything to do with "getting fit," it can be much easier to stick to a yoga practice. Because, ultimately, yoga has very little to do with our Western obsession with fitness; it's all about understanding our connection with the universe and detaching from the material obsessions of life. I know, this probably doesn't jive with the coconut-water-infused evangelical hustle of your friendly neighborhood yoga studio. But it's true. Once you disassociate your yoga practice from Western fitness mumbo jumbo, it may not seem like such a big deal to roll out your mat in the privacy of your own home.

Once you get there, find an online yoga studio that works for you. Even for seasoned yoga asana practitioners, online classes are a great option because they provide class flexibility and availability that far exceed the offerings of even the most yoga-friendly metropolises. For me, Yogaglo (yogaglo.com) is the perfect fit—with unlimited classes for less than twenty bucks a month, it's exponentially cheaper than drop-in rates at my local yoga studios, and the wide variety of instructors means I never get bored. There's always a new class to try, and they all constantly push my mental and physical boundaries.

Also, online classes are a great way to try out classes you might be a little *too* intimidated to attend in a live studio. For instance, Ashtanga yoga intimidated me for ages because of its extreme athleticism and the tendency of its instructors to be, shall we say, "verbally intense" with inexperienced practitioners. However, I found a great online class taught by the world-renowned Ashtanga teacher Kino MacGregor, and it fit my needs perfectly. In the safety and comfort of my own home, I'm able to try out one of the most challenging asana practices with an extremely skilled instructor. There are oodles of online yoga studios, so shop around.

WHAT YOGA GEAR DO YOU SPECIFICALLY RECOMMEND FOR CURVY STUDENTS?

If you're curvy bodied, having certain yoga gear on deck 24/7 will definitely make your life a lot more pleasant. However, not all yoga classes are taught with curvy bodies in mind. If you have a lot of belly, ass, or thigh action, blocks can make all the difference when trying to modify a bevy of yoga poses. There are examples of all the block modifications that will revolutionize your practice sprinkled throughout the asana section (starting on page 73).

Similarly, if you're very busty, you know there's absolutely nothing worse than being choked by your own cleavage while practicing yoga asana. Looping a "real" yoga strap (not a tie, sash, or one of the other DIY options I mentioned on page 50) across your chest above the bust line can help protect your neck and throat from a cleavage-suffocation situation.

Sometimes you may be in a yoga environment where there aren't any props. It might be a style of yoga that doesn't use props or a space that doesn't typically host yoga classes, like a park or library. In those situations, props are definitely available on a BYO situation, and you'll be very glad that you took the time to have your own supplies at the ready. If you own two yoga blocks and a yoga strap, you should be set for a lot of situations.

HELP! MY TEACHER IS MAKING ME FEEL VERY SELF-CONSCIOUS.

Okay, this is the thing about your teacher: She, he, or they are not mind readers. They don't know you're feeling uncomfortable. They don't know you would rather their attention be elsewhere. All they know is you are a student in their class, and they want to have an impact on your life.

However, there are things you can do to make your experience easier. For example, tell your instructor that they are making you uncomfortable. I'm serious. Just be straight up and honest. Maybe not in the middle of practice, but right at the beginning or end of a yoga class is an absolutely appropriate time to let your instructor know they need to adopt a more hands-off approach to your yoga practice. Otherwise, they'll just continue to make you and others feel uncomfortable.

If that doesn't work, just find a new class. There is no part of practicing yoga that requires you to accept emotional abuse at the hands of instructors. There isn't a one-size-fits-all approach to this stuff. Find a teacher and class that actually resonates for you.

WHAT IF I FART DURING CLASS?

Everyone farts. It's part of the human experience. Oh what, you think you're special because you might let it rip while your legs are spread wide open and you have breath flowing evenly from head to toe? You ain't special. That's just what happens. Try not to be embarrassed, because it's not a big deal. I doubt anyone would ever say anything, but if someone tries to make you feel bad, then that person is obviously a giant douche monkey asshole who thinks their shit don't stink. But their shit does stink. And it's not a big deal.

WHAT IF I'M SLOWER THAN EVERYONE ELSE?

You probably will be slower than everyone else. Don't stress yourself out about it. You'll get faster as time goes on. It might not happen quickly, but if you put in the time and energy you will DEFINITELY see progress.

WHAT TIME OF DAY SHOULD I PRACTICE YOGA?

In his seminal book *Light on Yoga*, B. K. S. Iyengar makes a great case for practicing either in the morning or in the evening. For example, he says that when you practice in the morning, you're preparing for a full day of action, and since you're full of determination and hope, it's a good idea to practice harder asana. I, however, think you should just practice *whenever the fuck you feel like it*. Seriously. Just fit it in whenever you can. Examples of perfect times to practice yoga:

- 10 minutes of Iyengarian alignment work while waiting for your kids to get out of Cub Scouts

- 45 minutes of an online Jivamukti-style class in the basement of your office building

- 20 minutes of yin yoga holds on the floor next to your bed right before dozing off for the night

- 30 minutes of an Anusara YouTube class in your dorm room before class

- 90-minute Kundalini hot flow on a Saturday morning in your favorite studio

In my opinion, it doesn't matter what time you practice, as long as you *do* practice. Don't hem yourself in, don't guilt yourself for being a busy person, and don't try to change who you are—accept the weirdness of your life, and build a yoga practice around it.

Furthermore, if for some reason you ever take a break from or *stop* practicing yoga, DON'T STRESS OUT ABOUT IT. Seriously. Yoga hiatuses happen to the best of us—they still happen to me from time to time. Shit happens, life gets crazy, and you start making excuses to not practice. Just remind yourself that it's really okay—there isn't a grand yoga scorekeeper who's going to dock points or humiliate you. The practice is always there whenever you're ready to return.

WHAT IF I'M THE <u>FATTEST</u>[13] PERSON IN CLASS AND EVERYONE STARES AT ME?

Look, before we go even a step further, let me just answer your question with a question: "Who Cares?" You heard me. Who cares? Who cares if people stare at you? What difference does it make in the long run? Stop adjusting yourself to fit the desires of others—you're perfect as you are, right now. In this exact moment. Yoga is probably one of the better ways to combat these emotions—as your spirit is strengthened by the practice, it will become easier to tune out the white noise of other people's judgments. However, I can't lie—this is no easy feat. I can't deny that I still find it frustrating to have my practice scrutinized by others, especially when it's ostensibly because of my size.

At the end of the day, the only reason we're bothered by people who shamelessly stare is our assumption that staring means we are doing something wrong. It's extremely common for anyone who presents themselves in a way that contradicts societal norms to be stared at by people who strive to present themselves in a socially acceptable way. That doesn't mean you're doing anything wrong.

If someone is staring at you with disgust or anger on their face, remember that they are probably melting under a host of body issues which they've decided to project onto you. The best response in this situation is an even mix of compassion toward the other person paired with an attitude of "suck it"—frankly, you don't need someone else's self-hate fucking up your chance to get lifted. In many ways, learning to distract ourselves from the projected emotions of others is an excellent expression of the eight-limbed path, particularly the limb of Pratyahara (page 38) and the niyama of Svadhyaya (page 37). Use your yoga practice as a vehicle to disregard the opinions of others—once you solidify this attitude on your yoga mat, you'll be able to maintain it off your mat as well.

---

13 For the record, I am only using the word "fat" as a placeholder—we each have some kind of drama with our physical body that we think inhibits our path toward perfection. If you don't consider yourself to be "fat," just insert your bullshit body baggage here.

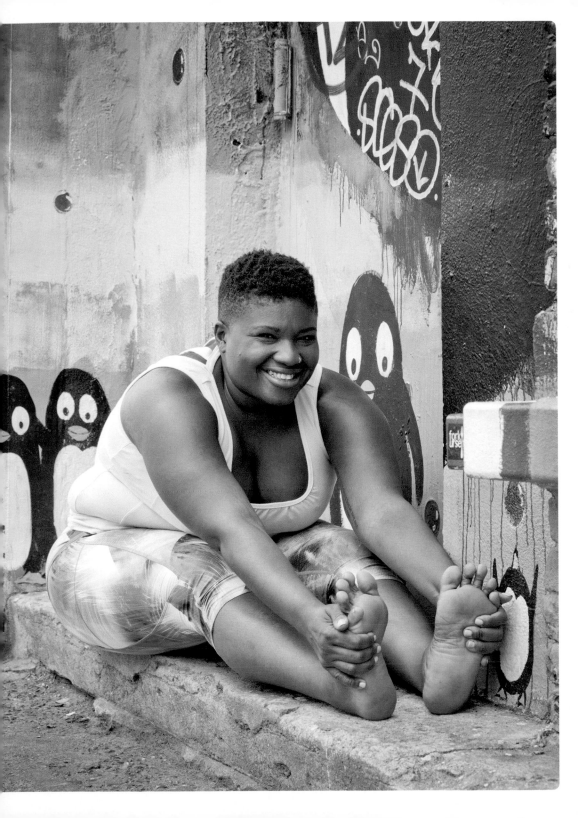

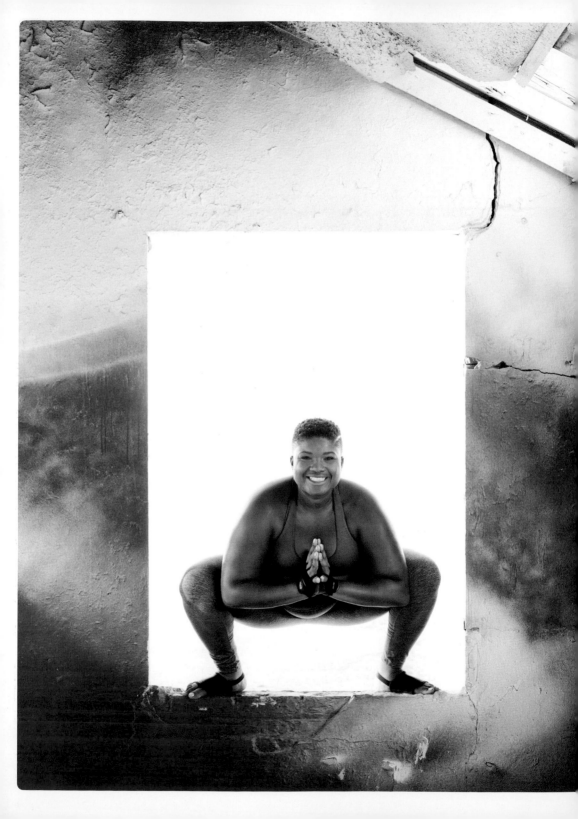

PART 3

Jessamyn's ABCs of Asana

GETTING STARTED WITH ASANA

What follows are the poses that make up the foundation of my own yoga arsenal—in my mind, they are the "ABCs of asana." I call them ABCs because learning these poses was a lot like learning a basic yoga alphabet or vocabulary. Once the poses become more familiar, we're able to weave them into flow sequences that resemble a dense and informative body language. When I began practicing asana, these were the poses that drew me under the spell of yoga. I would spend days, weeks, months, and (eventually) years falling down, learning new things about my body, and trying to breathe all at the same time. The asana are divided into categories based upon bodily action and which part of the body is particularly emphasized—poses are either standing, balance, core, hips, hamstrings, backbends, or restorative. But don't fool yourself into thinking these are the only poses available to you—these are merely the tip of the iceberg.

Before I get to the asana poses, let's work through the nuts and bolts of an asana practice to ensure that you have a strong, safe experience on the mat.

"WHAT DO I DO WHEN I ROLL OUT MY YOGA MAT?"

When you roll out your yoga mat, pretend like there's a straight line down the middle of your mat. This line symbolizes the internal midline of your body, which is essentially your body's internal compass. When you practice making any asana shapes on your yoga mat, think about pulling your bodily attention into this internal midline.

When placing your hands and feet upon the mat, think about pouring all of your energy evenly through your toes, heels, balls of the feet, fingertips, and knuckles. Avoid placing all of your weight solely upon your wrist or ankle joints—when weight and energy are poured evenly through all four corners of the feet and hands, it's possible to stand strong and find balance in a myriad of different shapes.

"OK, I'M ON MY MAT . . . NOW WHAT?"

Begin every yoga practice with a few minutes of quiet Pranayama breath work—this will center your energy and help allow you to draw your focus solely on your yoga mat. You can utilize any of the methods found on the next page, but allow this to become the most important part of your practice.

Breathing is arguably the most underestimated and underrated aspect of the modern yoga practice. Pranayama (page 37) takes its name from prana, the cosmic energy that exists within all living creatures and the world around us. In essence, prana is the connective energy that draws all living beings together. By breathing, we draw prana into our own bodies as self-sustenance on an inhale and then release prana as sustenance to others on the exhale. When done properly, breath work can elevate a standard yoga asana practice to a place of prayer and devotion—and provide endless relief in moments of life stress and duress.

Yogic philosophy indicates that breath should always come before motion—in essence, taking a breath should precede and guide all action. This is true for our lives both on and off the mat. When a yoga student feels as though they may die during class, it's usually because they've forgotten to breathe. The breath is typically the first thing to go when we start to stress out in life, too—panic attacks and anxiety attacks are often brought about by an insufficient amount of oxygen. First goes breath, then goes focus, and before long your face is beet red and your ass is in a heap on the floor. However, by allowing the breath to become the primary focus of any yoga practice, practitioners are able to sustain longer and more physically arduous asana, as well as progress to more complex and advanced pose variations. When we breathe consciously, actively, and deeply, the constant exchange of prana creates an opportunity for greater union with the world around us.

Before starting an asana practice, it's always nice to begin with a few rounds of deep breathing—it anchors physical and mental action, while providing a point of focus for the rest of the practice. In my experience, devoting at least 5 to 10 minutes to the establishment of powerful breath works.

Here are two of my favorite ways to practice pranayama:

TYPE	HOW DO YOU DO IT?	WHEN SHOULD I BREATHE LIKE THIS?
Ujjayi breath (victorious breath)	Close your eyes and breathe in through your nose, out through your nose—but keep your mouth shut.	During all types of flow yoga, especially vinyasa styles. Before any movement, it's a great idea to sit or stand quietly with the eyes closed and establish a strong ujjayi breath as a source of recurring energy for the practice as a whole.
Alternate nostril breathing	Close your eyes. Using your right hand, close off the right nostril with the thumb and inhale through your left nostril. Then close your left nostril with your fourth finger and exhale fully through your right nostril. Inhale again through your right nostril. Close the right nostril and exhale fully through your left.	This is a great way to begin or end a practice, or to kick off a meditation practice.

"OK, I'VE ESTABLISHED MY BREATH AND I'M FEELING MUCH MORE RELAXED. WHAT'S NEXT?"

After breath work, move into a fairly primal warm-up sequence, moving through poses like Cat/Cow Pose (page 114) and Extended Puppy Dog Pose (page 115) to help wake up your spine, joints, and muscles. This warm-up is key, especially if you're practicing yoga immediately after waking from slumber.

"BUT THEN WHAT DO I DO AFTER WARMING UP? I THOUGHT YOU SAID YOGA WOULD KICK MY ASS!"

Adding Sun Salutations (pages 144 and 148) after a warm-up is a great way to invite heat and energy into the body. You can "flow" or link the individual poses together using your ujjayi breath (page 65), and I like to hold each Sun Salutation pose for 1 to 3 breaths each. Some practitioners prefer to hold each Sun Salutation pose for only 1 breath, but to each their own.

"OK, THOSE SUN SALUTATIONS REALLY HYPED ME UP—HOW DO I CONNECT THE DOTS TO THE REST OF MY HOME PRACTICE?"

After Sun Salutations, I like to mix and match pose sequencing by directing focus toward specific bodily areas so that my entire body becomes more open and limber. Think about adding an even mix of standing and seated postures, as well as an even mix of different body areas. Usually, I practice poses in this order: standing (page 74), balance (page 88), hamstrings and core (page 94), hips (page 104), backbends (page 114), and restorative (page 124)—however, don't be afraid to mix poses together in unexpected ways to create the best medicine for your body.

There are times when you may read an instructional cue, try to do it at home, and not see a visual change in your body. That doesn't mean you're practicing the pose incorrectly—not all instructional cues will make an immediate visual difference in your body. It's all about feeling your way through the asana into your personal variation of each pose.

I USE SOME YOGA LINGO IN THIS TEXT THAT MIGHT BE A LITTLE STRANGE IF YOU'RE SEEING IT FOR THE FIRST TIME. IF YOU GET CONFUSED WHILE LEARNING THE POSES IN THIS BOOK, REFER TO THIS GLOSSARY TO HELP CLARIFY THINGS:

"Activate"—to ignite with energy

"Claw" or "Plug"—to plant the fingertips or toes into the mat very aggressively, much like how other animals dig their claws into the earth

"Corset"—to pull in and tighten, like tightening the strings of a whalebone corset.

"Gaze"—(v): to direct your eyesight with focus and concentration; (n): a point of focus, also known as "drishti" in Sanskrit

"Melt"—to relax

"Pump"—to draw out, up, and forward, like pumping water out of a well

"Soften"— to release tension

"Spiral"—to twist

"Root"—to anchor your body parts to the ground and allow energy to flow

"Wrap"—to rotate inward

HOW LONG SHOULD I HOLD A POSE?

Some schools of yoga call for very specific pose holds—Ashtanga yoga (page 42), for example, specifically calls for five deep breaths per pose. However, in a world of "build your own yoga," I think it should be left to the discretion of the practitioner. In my own practice, I typically like to aim for between 3 and 5 breaths per pose. If I'm working on core-heavy poses like High Plank Pose (page 94) or Dolphin Pose (page 99), I think it's fun to challenge my body by holding the poses for 5 to 10 breaths each. Listen to your body, and don't be afraid to challenge yourself—each breath is an opportunity to breathe additional space into your body. Listen to the rhythm, and be your own teacher.

OK, I THINK I'VE GOT THE IDEA. BUT HOW DO I PULL MY HOME YOGA SEQUENCES TOGETHER?

I've offered some sequence suggestions in Part 4 (page 137), and these sequences will provide inspiration as you start to create sequencing of your very own. It's a good rule of thumb to practice each sequence twice—once on each side of your body, right and left.

When I "flow" yoga poses together in a sequence, I like to hold each pose for 3 to 5 breaths each, challenging myself to relax into the shapes for as long as possible while internalizing new anatomical cues in my body.

When using yoga blocks in supported poses like Standing Half Forward Fold (page 78), try not to bear *all* of your weight into the props. Simply use the blocks to help balance weight throughout your *entire* body.

After completing a given sequence on one leg or "side" of my body, I like to take a "vinyasa" before switching to the second leg or "side." (See page 167.)

Sometimes, yoga sequencing may kick your ass in a way you're not expecting, and you may find it necessary to drop down to your knees and take a break. That's totally fine—don't beat yourself up about it. While you're taking a little break, close your eyes and just try to find your ujjayi breath again (page 65). Once you have your breath under control, it will be much easier to pick yourself back up and keep practicing.

Let your creativity shine through and allow your body to move intuitively—once you become familiar with the yoga poses in this book, you'll feel at ease linking the poses together in new ways.

"SO THESE ARE GOOD TIPS, BUT HOW WILL I KNOW THAT I'M ACTUALLY PRACTICING THESE POSES CORRECTLY AND SAFELY WITHOUT AN INSTRUCTOR WATCHING MY EVERY MOVE?"

I believe that my yoga practice began to take shape and really *mean* something when I began photographing my practice. I was apprehensive to turn the camera on myself—for one thing, I didn't like looking at my body. In the beginning, every time I took a yoga photo of myself I couldn't seem to do much but focus negative attention on all of my perceived flaws—chief among them being my gobble neck, my flabby arms, and my gelatinous belly fat.

But the more I practiced yoga in the comfort of my home, the easier it became to stop caring about the body parts I'd been taught to hate. And, as my confidence began to spike, I found it harder to nitpick at my body in yoga snapshots. I became impressed by the strength I was exhibiting in my poses. Unlike a reflection in a mirror, photographs freeze a moment in time. And there's something pretty magical about seeing a frozen moment in time wherein strength is unavoidable and can't be acknowledged as anything else. It's incredibly empowering in a way provided by very few other options.

If you have any perceived body discomfort, shame, or hate, I can't provide a strong enough recommendation for photographing your yoga asana practice. It's not about proving that you can "do" a pose—it's about creating an honest, loving dialogue with your body in which you stare at the body parts you've been taught to hate and instead coat them with love and adoration because of their undeniable strength and ability.

You don't have to use a fancy camera or acquire professional photography equipment—most of my best yoga photos have been taken with my cell phone's camera in dark corners of my living room. To this day, I maintain a fairly rudimentary yoga photography setup—my cell phone camera and a yoga block turned camera "tripod" are my only tools. It wouldn't hurt to consider investing in a remote control so you can take photos from a distance without hustling to and from the "tripod." Experiment with angles and lighting, and don't obsess over the final product—just enjoy the process of igniting your internal Diane Arbus.

SO HOW DO I LOOK?

I hate this question. Every day we ask ourselves and each other, "How do I look?" Echoing within homes, workplaces, and every space in between, the question "How do I look?" can dictate every type of life decision, from deciding what clothes to wear in the morning to determining what people, places, or jobs we deserve to pursue. This question has invaded yoga studios as well. Many potential yoga students may never even enter a classroom

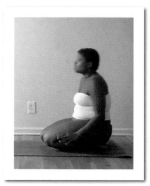 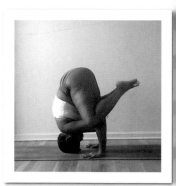 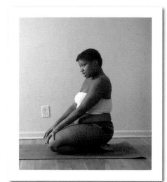

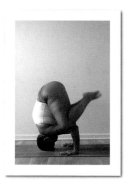 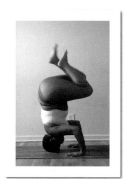 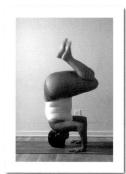 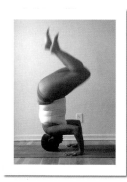

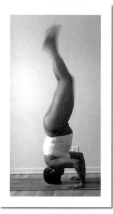 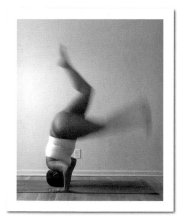 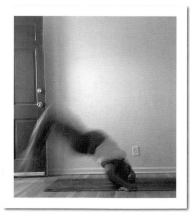

It's called a yoga <u>practice</u> for a reason. Don't strive for perfection. Don't be afraid to fall down—or laugh at yourself. Falling down is a crucial part of the process. Even in your "unsuccessful" asana photos, look for little alignment adjustments you can make in future asana attempts.

for fear of receiving a negative answer to "How do I look?" Even veteran students can be haunted by the question. I can't count the number of people who say they are certain they'll never be able to work on inversions, arm balances, or deep backbends simply because of the way their bodies look.

Yoga students belittle their practices by constantly asking, "How do I look?" Yoga is not about physical appearance. It's about self-discovery—it's about realigning with your true self. So instead of asking, "How do I look?" when practicing yoga, always ask yourself, "How do I feel?" When bending deeply in a Warrior Pose, don't think about how your body appears physically. Ask, "How do I feel?" Do your feet feel firmly rooted in the ground? Do your hips feel square? Does your weight feel evenly distributed? Are you feeling fire in your quads? These are the questions that actually matter—these are the questions you should actively try to answer. If your answer to "How do I feel?" is "NOT GOOD," you will be much better equipped to strengthen your yoga practice than you would be with the answer to "How do I look?"

By speaking of ourselves in a positive and affirmative fashion and finding ways to eradicate self-hate, by speaking kindly about ourselves and those around us, we can foster a sense of love and compassion powerful enough to restructure our society's entire perspective of "body love." In many ways, by speaking kindly about our bodies and those around us, we engage in the Yama of Ahimsa (page 36) and are able to walk further along the eight-limbed path of yoga (page 35). And when we restructure the general perspective of body love, we are able to make space in our society for new definitions of powerful beauty.

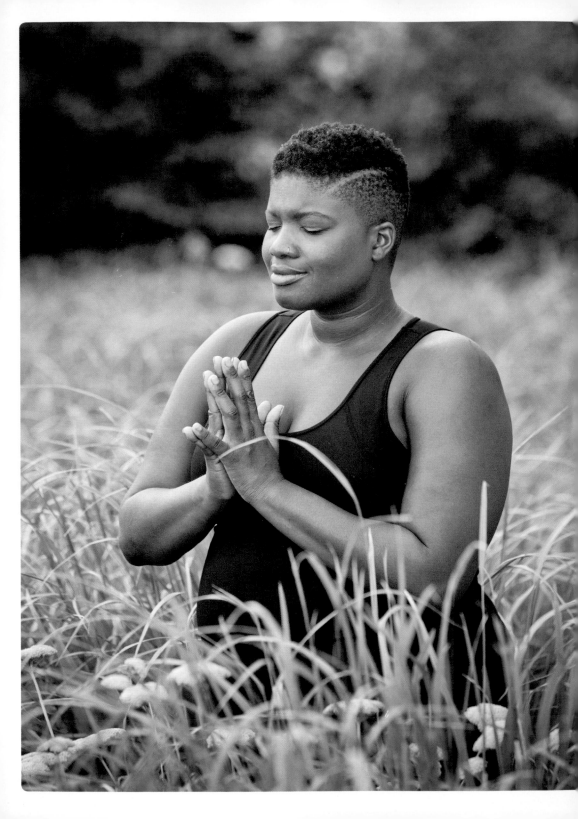

THE POSES

MOUNTAIN POSE
Tadasana

- Stand tall, toes pointing forward either hip width apart or with your feet together and with big toes touching.

- Distribute your weight evenly through all four corners of your feet.

- Relax your shoulders, lengthen your neck, and let your arms relax at your sides. Look straight ahead and soften your gaze, allowing your facial muscles to relax.

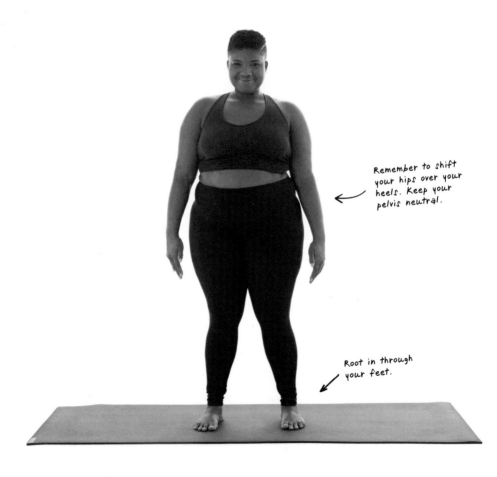

Remember to shift your hips over your heels. Keep your pelvis neutral.

Root in through your feet.

UPWARD SALUTE

Urdhva Hastasana

- Begin in Mountain Pose (page 74). On an inhale, raise your arms above your head with palms facing each other.

- Stretch long and tall through your arms and fingers, extend your inner elbows, and draw your shoulder blades toward each other.

- Keep your neck soft, releasing all tension, and feel the stretch along both sides of your body.

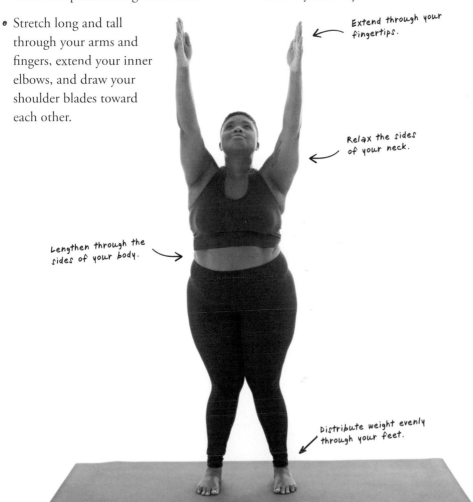

Extend through your fingertips.

Relax the sides of your neck.

Lengthen through the sides of your body.

Distribute weight evenly through your feet.

STANDING FORWARD FOLD

Uttanasana

- Start in Mountain Pose (page 74), feet hip-width apart. Inhale, lifting your arms up into Upward Salute (page 75), and stretch through your fingertips to extend through the sides of your body.

- On the exhale, fold forward from your hips as you draw your arms, hands, and heart to the floor.

- Actively shift your hips to the sky and rock the weight back into your heels so that your hips, knees, and ankles are in one line.

- A bend in your knees will help you lengthen through your lower back and hamstrings.

- Release all effort and encourage your body to relax and soften. When you're ready, with a flat back, lift your arms and rise back into Mountain Pose.

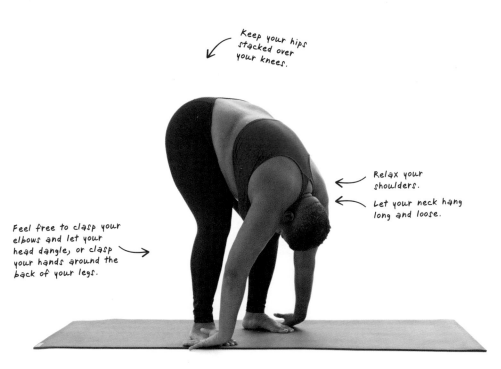

Keep your hips stacked over your knees.

Relax your shoulders.

Let your neck hang long and loose.

Feel free to clasp your elbows and let your head dangle, or clasp your hands around the back of your legs.

VARIATION: *BIG TOE HOLD* Padangusthasana

- Start in Mountain Pose, feet hip-width apart. Inhale as you lift your arms into Upward Salute and, on the exhale, fold forward from your hips and grip your big toes between your thumbs and first two fingers.

- Send your tailbone and pelvis to the sky on an inhale and, on an exhale, draw your head toward your knees by pulling your toes for leverage without lifting them off the floor. After a few breaths, release your toes and rise back to Mountain Pose.

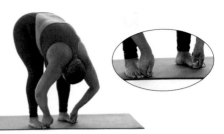

VARIATION: *HAND UNDER FOOT* Padahastasana

- Start in Mountain Pose, feet hip-width apart. Inhale, while lifting your arms into Upward Salute and, on the exhale, fold forward from your hips and slide your hands under your feet—you want your palms touching the soles of your feet.

- Send your tailbone and pelvis to the sky on an inhale and, on an exhale, draw your head toward your knees by bending your elbows and pulling against your feet using the palms. After a few breaths, slide your hands out and rise back to Mountain Pose.

STANDING HALF FORWARD FOLD
Ardha Uttanasana

UNSUPPORTED

- Start in Standing Forward Fold (page 76) and, on an inhale, walk your fingertips forward to extend your spine, chest, and gaze forward. You may not need to walk your fingertips forward in order to feel your spine lengthen, but if you have a belly like mine, feel free to walk your hands forward.

- Allow your spine to lengthen and any tension in your upper back to melt as your heart draws forward.

- On an exhale, fold forward and return to Standing Forward Fold.

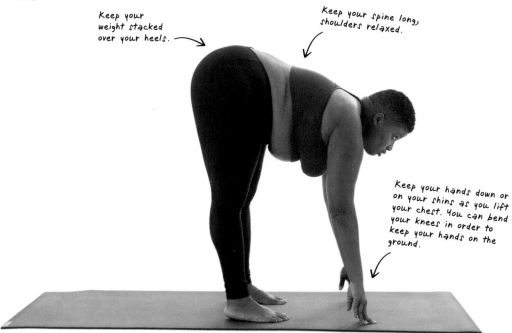

Keep your weight stacked over your heels.

Keep your spine long, shoulders relaxed.

Keep your hands down or on your shins as you lift your chest. You can bend your knees in order to keep your hands on the ground.

SUPPORTED

Props: 2 blocks

- Start in Standing Forward Fold and, on an inhale, walk your fingertips forward and place your hands on blocks at the tall or medium level, depending on your body. Extend your spine, chest, and gaze forward.

- Allow your spine to lengthen and any tension in your upper back to melt as your heart draws forward.

- On an exhale, fold forward and return to Standing Forward Fold.

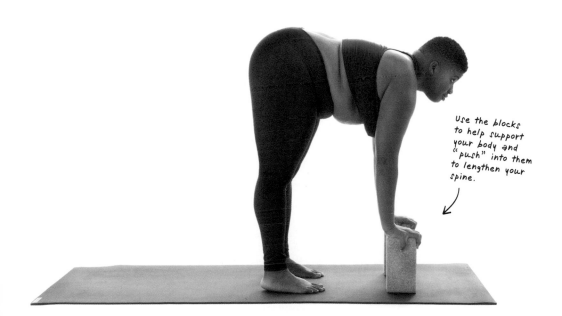

Use the blocks to help support your body and "push" into them to lengthen your spine.

DOWNWARD-FACING DOG
Adho Mukha Svanasana

UNSUPPORTED

- Begin on your hands and knees with your arms straight, your shoulders stacked over your wrists, and your hips stacked over your knees.

- Walk your hands about 6 inches ahead of your shoulders, curl your toes under, and lift your hips.

- Put a bend in your knees, drawing your chest toward your thighs. Walk forward, straightening your legs by pushing into your palms and lifting your hips up and back.

- Spread your fingers wide, distributing the weight evenly through your hands. Keep your arms straight with hands shoulder-distance apart, rotating your outer upper arms in, broadening across the shoulder blades and corseting your ribs inward.

- Press the tops of your thighs back while drawing the heels of your feet away from your toes, gradually guiding your heels toward the floor.

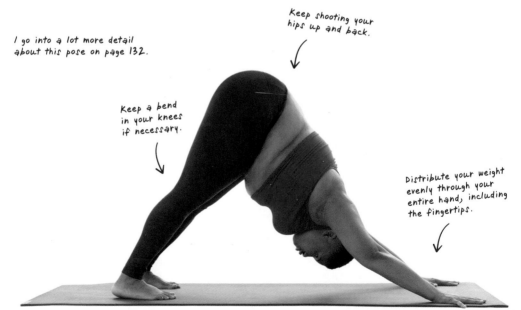

Keep shooting your hips up and back.

I go into a lot more detail about this pose on page 132.

Keep a bend in your knees if necessary.

Distribute your weight evenly through your entire hand, including the fingertips.

SUPPORTED

Props: 2 blocks

Note: This variation is particularly good for people with weak wrists.

- Begin on all fours with your arms straight, your shoulders stacked over your wrists, and your hips stacked over your knees.

- Place your hands on the blocks, just ahead of your shoulders. Curl your toes under and lift your hips.

- Use the blocks as a weight stabilizer, helping you find a balance between the top and bottom halves of your body.

- Work toward straightening your legs by pushing into your palms and shooting your hips up and back.

- Spread your fingers wide, distributing the weight evenly through your hands. Keep your arms straight, rotating your outer upper arms in, broadening across the shoulder blades, and corseting in your ribs.

- Press the tops of your thighs back while drawing the heels of your feet away from your toes, gradually guiding your heels toward the ground.

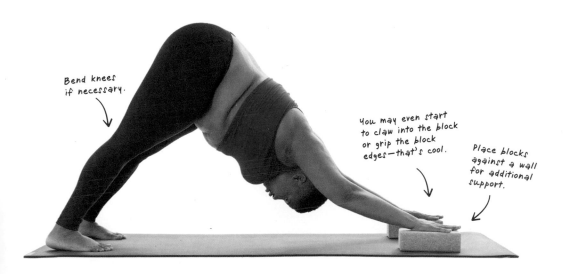

Bend knees if necessary.

You may even start to claw into the block or grip the block edges—that's cool.

Place blocks against a wall for additional support.

CHAIR POSE

Utkatasana

- Start in Mountain Pose (page 74) with your feet together or hip-width apart.

- Bend your knees and let your hips drop—as if sitting in a chair—with the weight coming into your heels.

- Draw your ribs into the midline of your body and sweep your arms up, shoulder-width apart. Keep shifting your lower legs back so you can still see your toes. Keep your shoulders relaxed and gaze skyward.

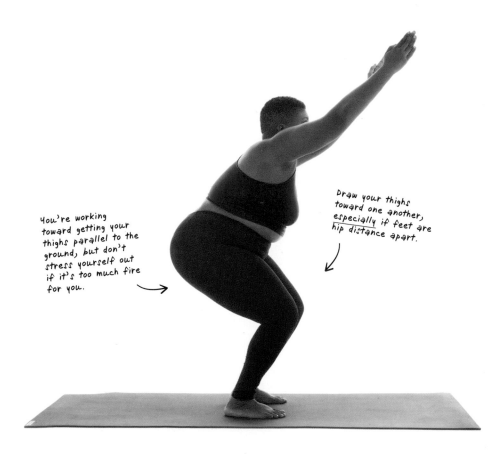

You're working toward getting your thighs parallel to the ground, but don't stress yourself out if it's too much fire for you.

Draw your thighs toward one another, especially if feet are hip distance apart.

WARRIOR I
Virabhadrasana I

- Start in Mountain Pose (page 74) with your feet hip-width apart. Step one foot back about one leg length and turn your back foot so it is at a 45-degree angle to the back edge of the mat. Keep your front foot parallel with the side of the mat. Your heels should line up.

- Square your hips forward and bend into your front knee until your thigh is parallel with the floor. Try to get your front knee and ankle to stack on top of each other.

- Keeping your back leg straight, sink your pelvis toward the floor, and sweep your arms straight up to the sky. Take a few breaths, then step your rear leg forward to meet your front leg and return to Mountain Pose. Switch to the opposite side.

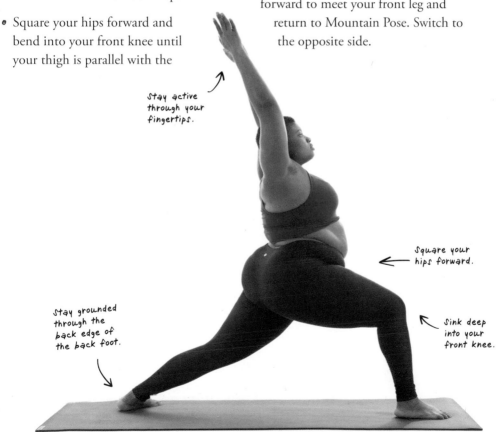

Stay active through your fingertips.

Square your hips forward.

Stay grounded through the back edge of the back foot.

Sink deep into your front knee.

WARRIOR II
Virabhadrasana II

- Start with your feet one leg length from each other. Rotate your front foot so it's parallel with the long edge of your mat and rotate your back foot so it's parallel with the short edge of your mat.

- Line up your front heel with your back foot's arch and bend deeply into your front knee so it lines up with your ankle (or as close as possible). You're trying to get your front thigh parallel to the ground—eventually. You may need to slide your front foot forward for this to happen.

- Try to keep your torso and pelvis neutral and stable, while corseting your ribs inward. Extend your arms until they are parallel to the floor with palms facing down. Gaze forward over your front fingers.

- Press into your front big toe and extend through your fingertips. Stay for a few breaths then straighten your front knee, turn your feet parallel with each other, and switch to the opposite side.

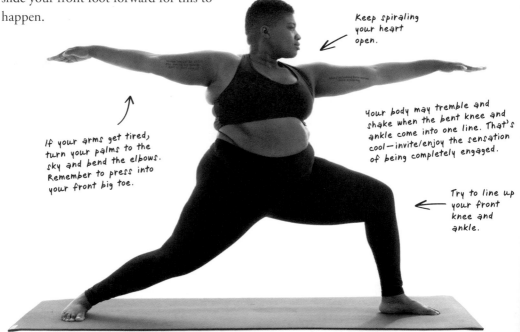

Keep spiraling your heart open.

If your arms get tired, turn your palms to the sky and bend the elbows. Remember to press into your front big toe.

Your body may tremble and shake when the bent knee and ankle come into one line. That's cool—invite/enjoy the sensation of being completely engaged.

Try to line up your front knee and ankle.

WARRIOR III

Virabhadrasana III

- Starting in Warrior I (page 83), shift your weight forward over your front leg and extend your back leg off the floor until it is parallel (or something like it) to the ground.

- Flex VERY actively through all ten of your toes, pressing into the big toe of your standing leg. Square your hips forward and spin your back toes to the floor or as close as possible.

- Gaze forward about 6 to 8 inches ahead of you on the ground and, if you're really feelin' it, extend your arms straight ahead of you like Super(wo)man. Stay here for a few breaths, then step the back leg into Warrior I before switching sides.

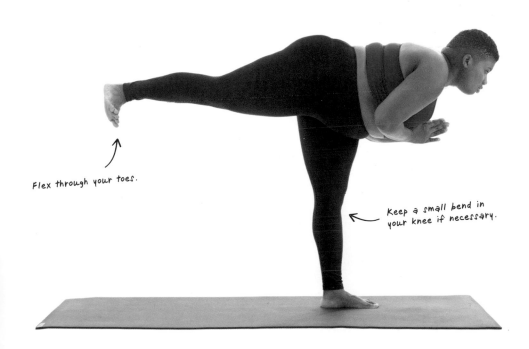

Flex through your toes.

Keep a small bend in your knee if necessary.

REVERSE WARRIOR POSE

Viparita Virabhadrasana

- Starting in Warrior II (page 84), keep your legs exactly as they are and sweep the palm of your front arm up and back while letting your rear hand touch your back thigh or calf.

- Spiral your torso open and stay for a few breaths, strengthening through your top fingers and opening your chest.

- Sweep your arms back into Warrior II, straighten your front knee and turn in your front foot so it's parallel with your back foot. Switch to the other side.

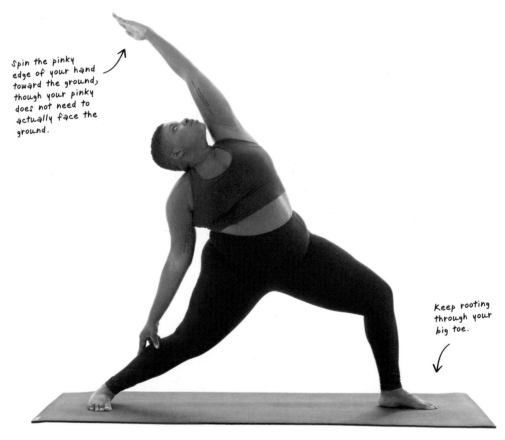

Spin the pinky edge of your hand toward the ground, though your pinky does not need to actually face the ground.

Keep rooting through your big toe.

EXTENDED TRIANGLE POSE
Utthita Trikonasana

UNSUPPORTED AND SUPPORTED
Optional Prop: 1 block

- Starting with your feet one leg length from each other, rotate your left foot out about 90 degrees and your right foot in about 45 degrees, but keep your heels in one line.

- Extend your arms over your legs until they are parallel to the floor and bring your left arm and hand down to your left shin, ankle, foot, or the ground. If using a block, put it on the inside or outside of your left shin and place your hand on it.

- Extend your right arm straight up to the sky and try to stack your shoulders.

- Roll your torso open and lengthen through your head to draw long through the sides of your body. Keep pulling your right hip away from your left toes. Stay for a few breaths, then switch sides.

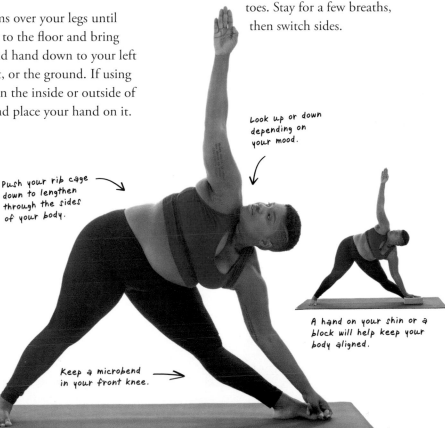

Look up or down depending on your mood.

Push your rib cage down to lengthen through the sides of your body.

A hand on your shin or a block will help keep your body aligned.

Keep a microbend in your front knee.

HALF MOON POSE
Ardha Chandrasana

SUPPORTED

Prop: 1 block

- From Extended Triangle Pose (supported, page 87), bring your right hand to your hip. Pick up your block with your left hand, bend your right knee, and transfer your weight over your right leg until your block rests on the ground about 8 inches ahead of your right toes.

- Kick your left leg up until it is close to parallel with the floor, flexing through the toes of your back foot.

- Shoot your left arm to the sky and try to stack your shoulders atop each other. Flex actively through all of your fingers and toes. Press into your bottom big toe to keep you balanced.

- If possible, try to look up along your raised arm. Stay for a few breaths (get back up even if you fall down), then switch sides.

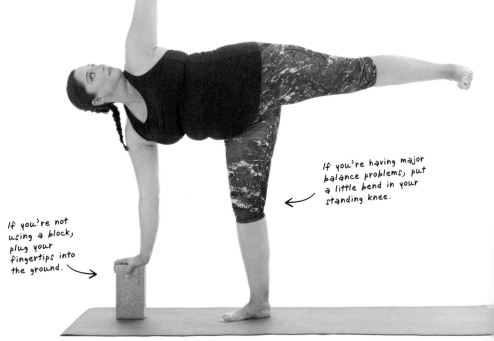

If you're having major balance problems, put a little bend in your standing knee.

If you're not using a block, plug your fingertips into the ground.

TREE POSE

Vrksasana

UNSUPPORTED AND SUPPORTED

Optional Prop: 1 block

- Starting in Mountain Pose (page 74), place a block next to your left ankle. Lift your left foot, bend the knee, and place your left toes on the block, with the ankle resting on your right leg. Pull in your hips toward your body's midline.

- If not using the block, lift your left foot, bend the knee, and draw the foot to your right ankle, mid-shin, or grab your inner left ankle and bring the sole of your foot to your right shin or upper thigh. Actively press your left foot and right leg into each other to maintain balance.

- Bring your palms to touch in front of your heart or extend your arms upward. Gaze forward or sweep your gaze up— you can even close your eyes. Stay for a few breaths, then switch sides.

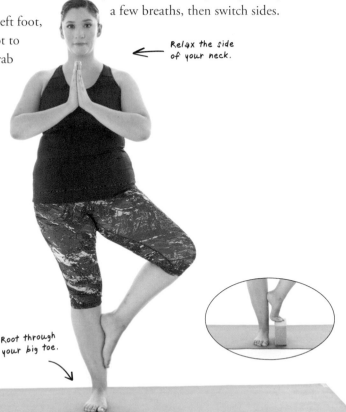

Relax the side of your neck.

Root through your big toe.

DANCER POSE
Natarajasana

SUPPORTED AND UNSUPPORTED

Optional Prop: 1 strap (make a loop with your strap that's big enough to hold your foot)

- Starting in Mountain Pose (page 74), place your right hand on your hip for balance and bend your left knee.

- Clasp the inside or outside of your left foot with your left hand and, using the power of your leg muscles, begin lifting your thigh.

- If using a strap, hold the strap in your left hand. With your right hand on your hip for balance, bend your left knee and place your foot into the strap. Hold the strap as close to your foot as you comfortably can.

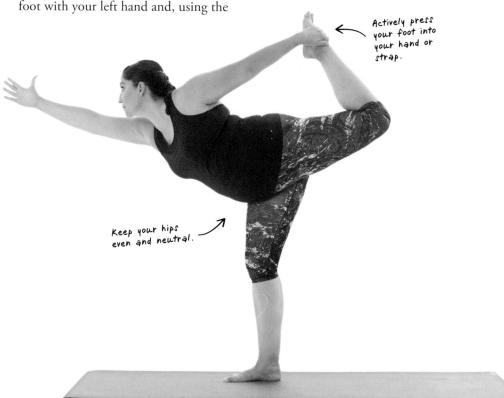

Actively press your foot into your hand or strap.

Keep your hips even and neutral.

- Keep squaring your hips forward and lifting your thigh away from the floor, actively flexing your foot into the hand or strap.

- Sweep your right arm forward and up, reaching through your fingers and still continuing to lift your thigh.

- Draw your standing thigh back and soften your heart forward. Stay for a few breaths, then switch sides.

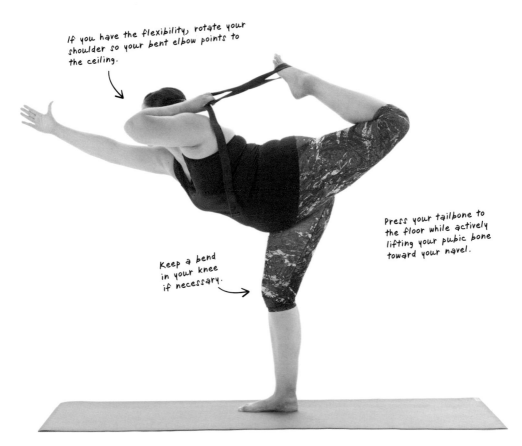

If you have the flexibility, rotate your shoulder so your bent elbow points to the ceiling.

Press your tailbone to the floor while actively lifting your pubic bone toward your navel.

Keep a bend in your knee if necessary.

EXTENDED HAND TO BIG TOE

Utthita Hasta Padangusthasana

UNSUPPORTED AND SUPPORTED

Optional Prop: 1 strap (make a loop with your strap that's big enough to hold your foot)

- Starting in Mountain Pose (page 74), bend your right knee toward your chest and hook your big toe with your right thumb and two forefingers.

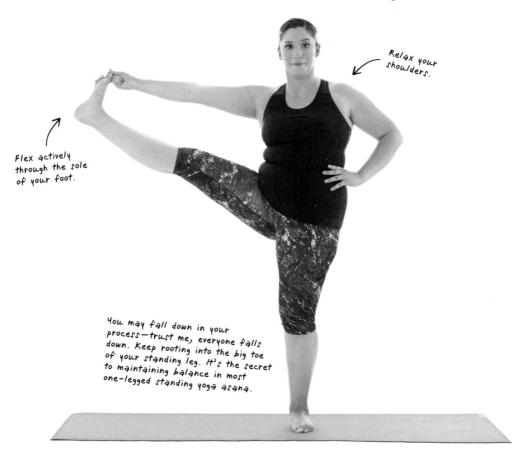

Relax your shoulders.

Flex actively through the sole of your foot.

You may fall down in your process—trust me, everyone falls down. Keep rooting into the big toe of your standing leg. It's the secret to maintaining balance in most one-legged standing yoga asana.

- If using a strap, bend your right knee and step your foot into the strap loop. Hold the strap as close to your foot as possible.

- With your left hand on your hip for additional balance, begin to extend your right leg straight out in front of you.

- Keep actively pressing into the big toe of your standing foot and relax your shoulders. Keep your hips even and shine your heart forward.

- Keep your gaze about 6 to 8 inches ahead of your toes on the ground and try to keep your standing leg straight. If you're feeling brave, look straight ahead or up to the sky.

- If you want, rotate your right hip out and continue raising your leg as you swing it out to the right side, keeping your hips level at all costs. Stay for a few breaths, then switch sides.

HIGH PLANK

Utthita Chaturanga Dandasana

UNMODIFIED

- Begin on all fours with your arms straight, your shoulders stacked over your wrists, and your hips stacked over your knees.

- Spread your weight evenly through your hands and grip your fingertips into the mat.

- Curl your toes under and step both of your legs straight back and hip-width apart. Stay on the balls of your feet,

with the core lifted and shoulders engaged. As your core lifts and your shoulders round, your hips may lift as well.

- Spread your fingers wide, distributing your weight evenly through your hands. Gaze beyond the fingertips. Wrap your outer upper arms in and extend your chest forward. Stay for a few breaths, then return to all fours.

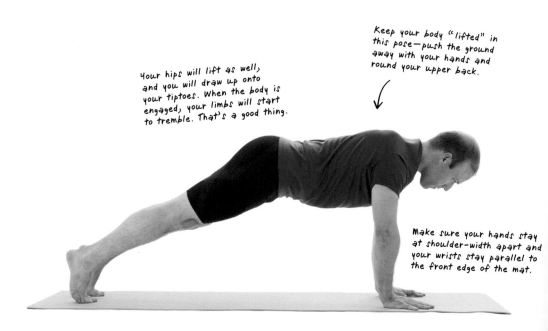

Keep your body "lifted" in this pose—push the ground away with your hands and round your upper back.

Your hips will lift as well, and you will draw up onto your tiptoes. When the body is engaged, your limbs will start to tremble. That's a good thing.

Make sure your hands stay at shoulder-width apart and your wrists stay parallel to the front edge of the mat.

MODIFIED (aka Tabletop Pose)

- Begin on all fours with your arms straight, your shoulders stacked over your wrists, and your hips stacked over your knees.

- Spread your fingers wide, distributing the weight evenly through your hands.

- Gaze beyond your fingertips. Firm your outer upper arms and release your neck to extend your chest.

- Work toward curling your toes and slowly stepping your legs straight into High Plank. Stay for a few breaths, then draw the hips back into Child's Pose (page 124).

Practice pushing the ground away with your hands and rounding your upper back. This will make you feel more sturdy and lifted, and will help prepare your body for unmodified High Plank.

Spread your fingers.

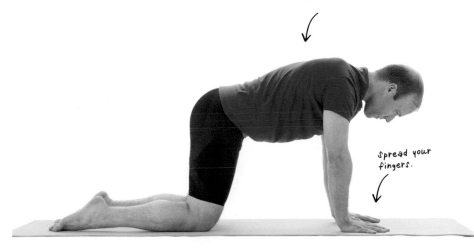

FOUR-LIMBED STAFF POSE

Chaturanga Dandasana

UNMODIFIED

• Begin in High Plank (page 94), extend your gaze forward, and engage your core in order to corset your front ribs in. Bend your elbows to 90-degree angles.

• Hug your elbows tight to your body and hover them over your wrists.

• Draw your shoulder blades down your back and extend your gaze forward. Stay for a breath (or a few breaths, depending on your mood) and then lower to your belly.

MODIFIED (aka "Half Chaturanga")

• Begin in High Plank, extend your gaze forward, and corset your front ribs in as you bend your elbows to 90-degree angles.

• Simultaneously drop your knees, chest, and chin toward the ground, stacking your elbows over your wrists.

• Keep your hips and shoulders in one line and engage your core.

• Draw your shoulder blades down your back, and extend your gaze forward. Stay for a breath (or a few breaths, depending on your mood) and lower to your belly.

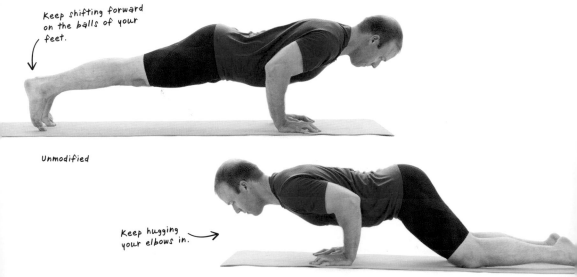

Keep shifting forward on the balls of your feet.

Unmodified

Keep hugging your elbows in.

Modified

WIDE-LEGGED FORWARD BEND

Prasarita Padottanasana

UNSUPPORTED

- Start with your feet parallel to each other, about 3 to 4 feet apart.

- With your hands on your hips, lengthen up through the crown of your head and put a bend in your knee. Hinge forward from your hips, letting your hands come to rest on the ground.

- Inhale your heart forward and straighten your arms, then exhale and fold forward over your legs. You can walk your hands back behind you, arms shoulder-distance apart, until your elbows bend into 90-degree angles, or you can hook your fingers around your big toes as in Big Toe Hold (page 77).

- Eventually, the crown of your head will reach the floor—however, it could be weeks, months, or years. In the meantime, keep sending your hips to the sky, and feel free to put a bend in your knees, much like in Standing Forward Fold (page 76).

- Stay for a few breaths, continuing to relax your shoulders, neck, and face at every opportunity. On an inhale, bring your hands back to the hips and slowly rise to your starting position.

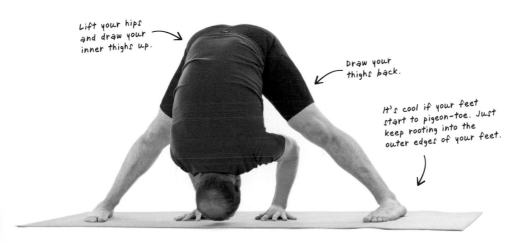

Lift your hips and draw your inner thighs up.

Draw your thighs back.

It's cool if your feet start to pigeon-toe. Just keep rooting into the outer edges of your feet.

Unsupported

SUPPORTED

Props: 1–2 blocks

- Start with your feet parallel to each other, about 3 to 4 feet apart. Place the block(s) at the tall or medium level between your legs.

- With your hands on your hips, lengthen up through the crown of your head. Hinge forward from your hips, letting your hands come to rest on the block(s).

- Inhale your heart forward and straighten your arms, then exhale and fold forward over your legs. If it's comfortable, let your hands come off the block(s) with palms flat on the ground. If *that* feels comfortable, walk them back between your legs as far as they will comfortably go.

- If you'd like, use one of your blocks to support your head. Let your head and neck relax on the block and work toward bending your elbows to 90 degrees with the arms shoulder-distance apart and palms flat on the ground. Tilt your pelvis down and send your hips up toward the sky. Feel free to put a bend in the knees, much like in Standing Forward Fold (page 76).

- Stay for a few breaths, relaxing your shoulders, neck, and face at every opportunity. On an inhale, bring your hands back to your hips and slowly rise to your starting position.

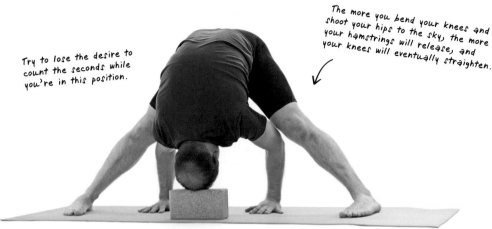

Try to lose the desire to count the seconds while you're in this position.

The more you bend your knees and shoot your hips to the sky, the more your hamstrings will release, and your knees will eventually straighten.

Supported

DOLPHIN POSE

Ardha Pincha Mayurasana

UNSUPPORTED

- Start in High Plank (page 94). Drop your forearms to the mat, shoulder-width apart. Plug into your fingertips and stack your shoulders over your elbows.

- On an inhale, lift your hips, straightening your legs as much as you can. This might be more than enough—if so, just chill here for a few breaths, then drop down to your knees.

- If you can, corset your front ribs in and walk forward toward your hands. Keep your shoulders over your elbows and relax your neck. Look slightly forward to your fingertips and try to walk so far forward that your hips line up over your shoulders.

- Start by trying to hold the pose for 3 to 5 breaths and then work up to holding it for 10 to 20 breaths. Take as many breaths as you need, then drop down to your knees and pull back into Child's Pose (page 124).

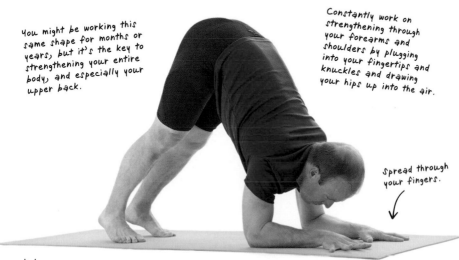

You might be working this same shape for months or years, but it's the key to strengthening your entire body, and especially your upper back.

Constantly work on strengthening through your forearms and shoulders by plugging into your fingertips and knuckles and drawing your hips up into the air.

Spread through your fingers.

Unsupported

SUPPORTED

Props: 1 block and 1 strap with a loop wide enough for your upper arms to slip in and stay braced at shoulder-distance apart

- Start in modified High Plank (page 95). With the strap resting just above your elbow joint and your arms shoulder-distance apart, drop your forearms to the mat, brace your hands on a block between your fingertips, and stack your shoulders over your elbows.

- On an inhale, curl your toes under and lift your hips, straightening your legs as much as you can. This might be more than enough—if so, just chill here for a few breaths, then drop down to your knees.

- If you can, corset your front ribs in and walk forward toward your hands. Keep your shoulders over your elbows and relax your neck. Grip the block for balance and press your outer arms into the strap.

- Look slightly forward to your fingertips and try to walk so far forward that your hips line up over your shoulders.

- Start by trying to hold the pose for 3 to 5 breaths and then work up to holding it for 10 to 20 breaths. You might be working this same shape for months or years, but it's the key to strengthening your entire body, and especially your upper back.

- Take as many breaths as you need, then drop down to your knees and pull back into Child's Pose (page 124).

- Claw the mat and try to plug into your fingertips and knuckles in order to strengthen your forearms and shoulders, all while drawing your hips up into the air.

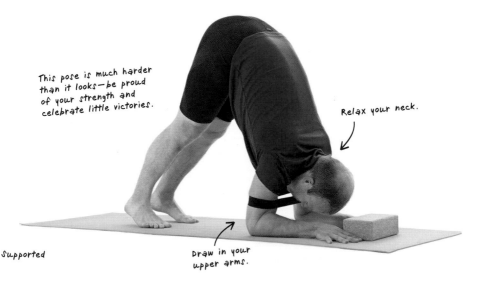

This pose is much harder than it looks—be proud of your strength and celebrate little victories.

Relax your neck.

Supported

Draw in your upper arms.

SUPPORTED HEADSTAND

Salamba Sirsasana

Note: Headstand is a challenging pose. It helps to divide it up into three stages: (1) getting your shoulders and head into position; (2) engaging your core and lifting up your legs; (3) finally settling into the inversion. The following instructions take you through each one of those phases. Move slowly and gradually. Master one at a time.

(1) SUPPORTED HEADSTAND PREP

- From modified High Plank (page 95), interlace your fingers and tuck your bottom pinky finger inside. Keep a space in your hands (NOT palms together) and put your hands on the ground.

- Place the crown of your head directly behind the heels of your hands and *cradle* your head without *holding* it.

- Curl your toes under, lift your knees, and walk your feet in toward your face as in Dolphin Pose (page 99). Stay here for as many breaths as you're able.

- Practice hugging your elbows in tight toward your head and pushing into your forearms so much that your shoulders become fully engaged and slightly rounded. In this shape, you should eventually be able to push into your forearms so much that your head can lift off the ground.

- After a few breaths, drop your knees to the floor and shift your hips back into Child's Pose (page 124).

(continued on next page)

Walk the feet in as close to the torso as possible.

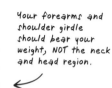

Your forearms and shoulder girdle should bear your weight, NOT the neck and head region.

(2) OPTION A: TUCK SHAPE

- Curl your toes under, lift your knees, and walk your feet in toward your face as in Dolphin Pose (page 99).

- Draw one knee in toward your chest and pull it in tightly. It may help to walk your legs out VERY wide beforehand. (This can be plenty of work; you might just stop here.)

- When you're ready, lightly hop your other foot in toward your chest so both knees are tucked in toward your chest. Tilt your pelvis so your hips start to come more in line with your shoulders and lift your knees to the sky. Flex your feet, draw your thighs together, and begin to flex your feet up to the sky.

- Continue lifting your shoulders and pressing your forearms into the ground. Lift your tailbone toward your toes, corset your ribs inward, and actively point and flex your toes.

- When you're ready, drop your legs back into a tuck shape and come down to your knees, drawing the hips back into Child's Pose (page 124).

(2) OPTION B: ONE-LEG LIFT

- Start in Supported Headstand (page 101).

- Curl your toes under, lift your knees, and walk your feet in toward your face as in Dolphin Pose (page 99).

- Reach one leg up to the sky and flex firmly through both hamstrings until the legs are pretty close to straight. Keep flexing through the toes of the top leg, scissor your thighs together, and flex the hamstring of the top leg so much that your pelvis tilts back and your bottom leg hovers off the ground.

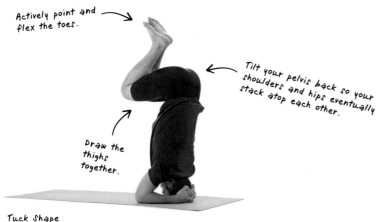

Actively point and flex the toes.

Tilt your pelvis back so your shoulders and hips eventually stack atop each other.

Draw the thighs together.

Tuck Shape

- Actively flex the feet of both legs and, if possible, bring your bottom leg up to meet your raised leg. Continue engaging your shoulders and pressing your forearms into the ground. Lift your tailbone toward your toes, corset your ribs inward, and actively point and flex your toes to keep your legs engaged with your body as a whole. When you're ready, drop your legs down individually and come down to your knees, drawing your hips back into Child's Pose (page 124).

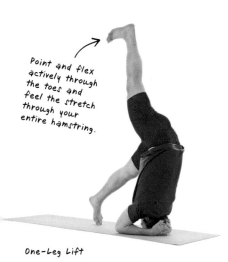

Point and flex actively through the toes and feel the stretch through your entire hamstring.

One-Leg Lift

(3) SUPPORTED HEADSTAND

Now we're going to pull it all together.

- Start in Supported Headstand Prep (page 101).

- Using either the Tuck Shape or the One-Leg Lift, draw your legs up to the sky, bearing your weight in your shoulders and pressing your forearms into the ground with minimal weight resting on your neck and head.

- Lift your tailbone toward your toes, pull your ribs inward, and point and flex your toes.

- Hold for 1 to 10 breaths and, when you're ready, drop your legs down individually or in a tuck shape and come down to your knees, drawing your hips back into Child's Pose (page 124).

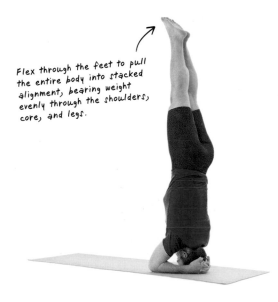

Flex through the feet to pull the entire body into stacked alignment, bearing weight evenly through the shoulders, core, and legs.

GARLAND POSE

Malasana

SUPPORTED AND UNSUPPORTED

Optional Props: 1–2 blocks and 1 blanket

- From Standing Forward Fold (page 76), walk your feet slightly wider than hip-width apart. If you have tender ankles or knees, slide a folded blanket longwise across your mat and rest your heels on the blanket.

- Spin your heels inward and your toes out, then sink your hips down into a low squat. If your hips are particularly tight or if you're finding the pose difficult, slide one or two blocks under your booty for added support.

- Snuggle both upper arms into your inner thighs and press your palms together to pump your heart forward.

- Stay for a few breaths, then return to Standing Forward Fold and shake out your hips. You've earned it.

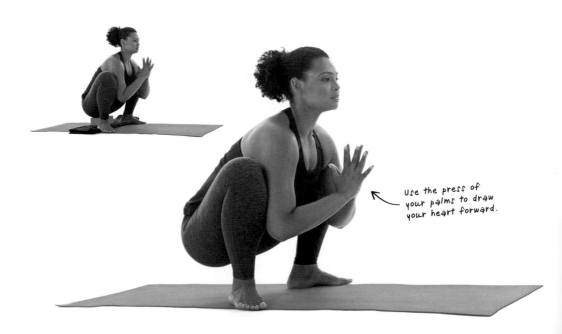

Use the press of your palms to draw your heart forward.

HIGH LUNGE POSE
Anjaneyasana

SUPPORTED AND UNSUPPORTED
Optional Props: 2 blocks

- From Downward-Facing Dog (page 80), exhale and step one foot forward between your hands, aligning your front knee over your heel at a 90-degree angle. If using blocks, place them at the medium or tall level on either side of your hips.

- Keep your back knee hovering above the floor and press into your front big toe, allowing the weight to distribute evenly through your front foot and the ball of your back foot.

- Inhale and lift your torso upright.

- Place your hands on blocks or on the ground, or sweep them to the sky.

- Keep drawing your tailbone toward your back heel, and pump your heart forward. Relax your neck and shoulders. Stay for a few breaths, and then switch sides.

Keep your hips level and your pelvis neutral.

Extend through your back heel.

 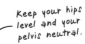

LOW LUNGE POSE

Anjaneyasana

SUPPORTED AND UNSUPPORTED

Optional Props: 2 blocks

- From Downward-Facing Dog (page 80), exhale and step one foot forward between your hands, aligning your front knee over your heel at a 90-degree angle.

- Lower your back knee to the floor. Press into the big toe of your front foot and allow the weight to distribute evenly though your front and back feet.

- With your front knee fixed in place, slide your knee back until you feel a comfortable stretch in your groin and your front thigh.

- Inhale and lift your torso upright with your hands on blocks, or on the ground, or sweep them to the sky.

- Drop your tailbone to the ground, slide your shoulder blades down your back, and pump your heart forward. Stay for a few breaths, and then switch sides.

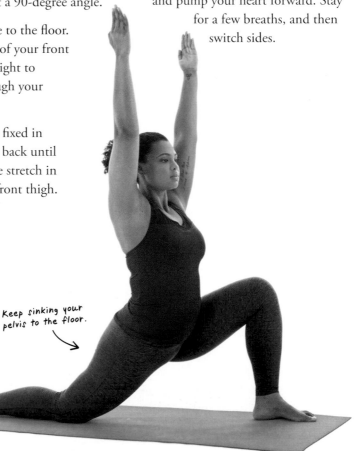

Keep sinking your pelvis to the floor.

LIZARD LUNGE POSE

Utthan Pristhasana

SUPPORTED AND UNSUPPORTED

Optional Props: 2 blocks

- From Downward-Facing Dog (page 80), step one foot forward between your hands to a lunge position.

- Bring both forearms to the floor inside your front leg.

- Inhale and lift your torso with your hands on blocks, or on the ground.

- Keep your back knee and inner thigh lifted and engaged, or drop your back knee to the ground. As your back heel reaches back, your heart pumps forward to create length in your upper back.

- Stay for a few breaths, and then switch sides.

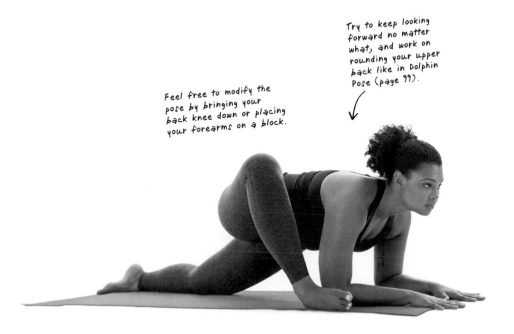

Try to keep looking forward no matter what, and work on rounding your upper back like in Dolphin Pose (page 99).

Feel free to modify the pose by bringing your back knee down or placing your forearms on a block.

RUNNER'S LUNGE

Hanumanasana (Prep)

SUPPORTED AND UNSUPPORTED

Optional Props: 2 blocks

- From Lizard Lunge Pose (page 107), with your knee on the mat, place both hands on the floor on either side of your front foot, and shift your hips back until your front leg is straight and your front toes point at the sky.

- Engage the muscles and knee joint of your front leg to protect the hamstring as you fold forward as far as you can while keeping your spine long and back flat.

- Place your hands on blocks or on the ground. Press down the top of the back foot and toes to help keep your tailbone long.

- Keep looking forward over your toes, relax your shoulders, pump your heart forward, and gaze over your front foot. Stay here for 5 to 10 breaths, and then switch sides.

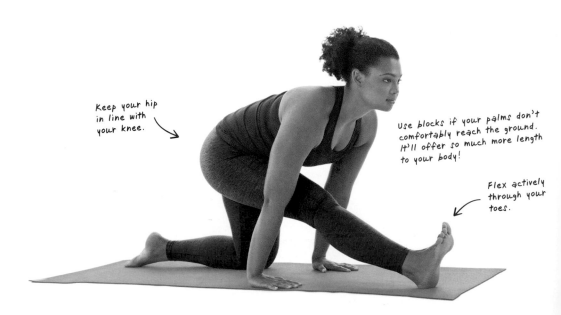

Keep your hip in line with your knee.

Use blocks if your palms don't comfortably reach the ground. It'll offer so much more length to your body!

Flex actively through your toes.

ONE-LEGGED KING PIGEON POSE

Eka Pada Rajakapotasana

UNSUPPORTED

- Come to High Plank (page 94) and draw your right knee to the floor near your hand and wrist. Bring your right foot to your opposite hip at a diagonal, with the outside of your right shin resting on the floor.

- Square your hips. Work on getting the edge of your front foot solidly on the ground, with the foot flexed and engaged.

- Slide your back foot toward the back edge of the mat and lower your thigh and groin to the floor. You can sit upright with your hands on the ground aligned with your shoulders, or you can fold forward over your front leg and relax your forehead on the ground. Relax your shoulders and steady your breath. Stay for several breaths, then switch sides.

(continued on next page)

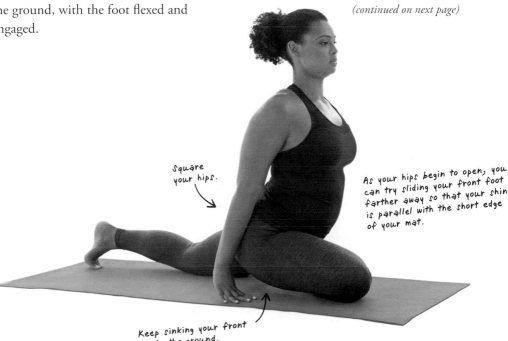

Square your hips.

As your hips begin to open, you can try sliding your front foot farther away so that your shin is parallel with the short edge of your mat.

Keep sinking your front hip to the ground.

SUPPORTED

Props: 1-3 blocks; bolster optional

- Come to modified High Plank (page 95) and draw your right knee forward to the floor near your hand and wrist. Bring your right foot to the opposite hip at a diagonal, with the outside of your right shin resting on the floor.

- Square your hips forward. As your hips begin to open, you can try sliding your front foot so that your shin is parallel with the short edge of your mat.

- Work on getting the edge of your front foot solidly on the ground with the foot flexed and engaged.

- Slide your back leg toward the back of the mat and lower your back thigh and groin to the floor. You can sit upright with your hands on the ground (or on blocks) aligned with your shoulders, or you can fold forward over your front leg and put your head on a block or bolster. Relax your shoulders and steady your breath. Stay for several breaths, then switch sides.

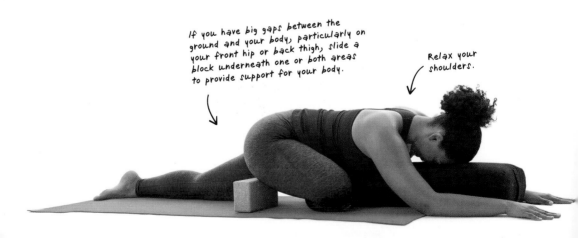

If you have big gaps between the ground and your body, particularly on your front hip or back thigh, slide a block underneath one or both areas to provide support for your body.

Relax your shoulders.

THREAD THE NEEDLE POSE

Sucirandhrasana

- Lie on your back with your knees pointing to the sky and your feet flat on the ground.

- Cross your left ankle over your right quad, just above the knee.

- Stick your left arm though the gap between your thighs and interlace your fingers just below your right knee or behind your right thigh.

- Draw your leg in toward your body until you feel significant sensation.

- If you want a little more stretch, stick your left elbow into your left thigh to intensify things. Stay for a few breaths, then switch sides.

Relax your shoulders to the floor—they want to get involved, but just tell them to chill out.

Keep shifting your hips toward the floor.

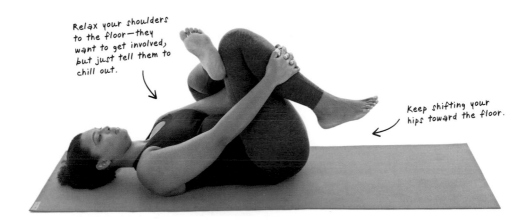

MONKEY POSE
Hanumanasana

UNSUPPORTED

- Start in Runner's Lunge (page 108) with your right leg forward and your hands on the ground.

- Wiggle your right leg forward until your thigh lowers to the ground, keeping the leg straight and the foot firmly flexed.

- Curl your back toes under, lift up your knee, and start sliding your foot as far back as possible. Keep wiggling and shimmying your front and back legs until your pelvis starts to descend to the ground. GO SLOWLY. Stop and take a few breaths before moving forward, and remember to actively point and flex your front toes.

- Try to square your hips, rolling your rear hip forward. Press your back toes firmly into the ground, and place your fingertips on the ground for support or sweep your arms up to the sky. Stay for a few breaths, then switch sides.

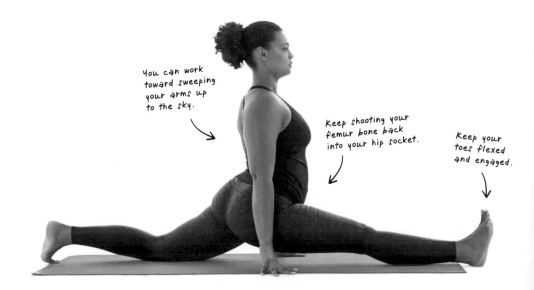

You can work toward sweeping your arms up to the sky.

Keep shooting your femur bone back into your hip socket.

Keep your toes flexed and engaged.

SUPPORTED

Props: 1–4 blocks (or more, if you want)

- Start in Runner's Lunge (page 108) with your right leg forward and your hands on blocks.

- Wiggle your right leg forward until your thigh lowers to the ground, keeping the leg straight and the foot firmly flexed.

- Curl your back toes under, lift up your knee, and start sliding your foot back as far as possible. Keep wiggling and shimmying your front and back legs

until your pelvis starts to descend to the ground. Keep your hands rooted on blocks for support and GO SLOWLY. Stop and take a few breaths before moving forward. Slide additional blocks under your front and back thighs if you want more support.

- Try to square your hips toward the front. Firm your right thighbone into its socket and engage your lower belly. Press your back toes firmly into the ground. Flex your front toes actively.

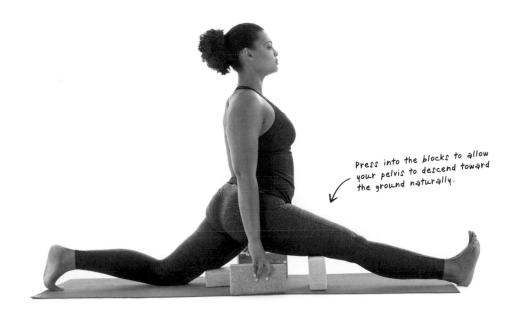

Press into the blocks to allow your pelvis to descend toward the ground naturally.

BACKBENDS
CAT/COW POSE
Marjaryasana/Bitilasana

- Begin in modified High Plank (page 95). On an inhale, keep your arms straight and drop your belly while rolling your shoulders back (Cow Pose). Extend and flex through your fingertips. Gaze up or forward.

- On an exhale, press into your hands and round your upper back while dropping your tailbone (Cat Pose).

- Plug into your fingertips and make the stretch dynamic—shake out your neck and head as you round your upper back and make faces to release tension in your jaw, ears, and eyes.

- Move between Cat and Cow until your spine is feeling loose and free.

- Remember to lower your belly on the inhale and round your spine on the exhale.

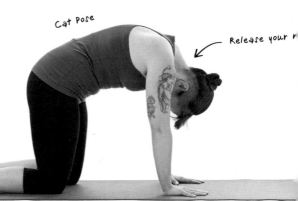

Cat Pose

Release your n

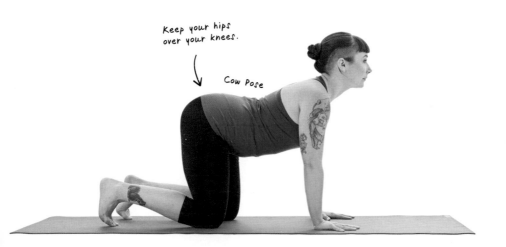

Keep your hips over your knees.

Cow Pose

EXTENDED PUPPY DOG POSE

Uttana Shishosana

- Starting in modified High Plank (page 95), keep your hips stacked over your knees and walk your arms out in front of you.

- Allow your belly, chest, and throat to melt toward the ground while wrapping your outer arms in and pressing into all ten toes.

- Keep your arms straight and relax your heart. Flex through your fingertips.

- Keep your gaze pointed forward the whole time. Stay for a few breaths, and then return to modified High Plank.

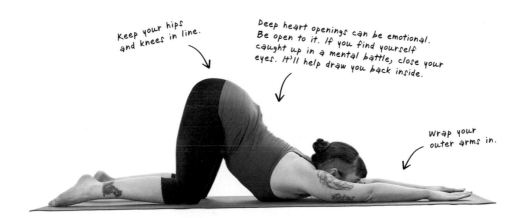

Keep your hips and knees in line.

Deep heart openings can be emotional. Be open to it. If you find yourself caught up in a mental battle, close your eyes. It'll help draw you back inside.

Wrap your outer arms in.

COBRA
Bhujangasana

- Begin on your belly with your legs hip-width apart, your palms flat on the floor next to your ribs, and your elbows just a touch ahead of your wrists.

- Press into your toes and engage your legs, rotate your inner thighs inward to broaden your lower back, and relax your butt muscles.

- On an inhale, press into your palms to lift your head and chest, drawing your ribs and belly off the floor. Keep your elbows bent, roll your shoulders back, and pull your heart through your arms. Gaze up and forward.

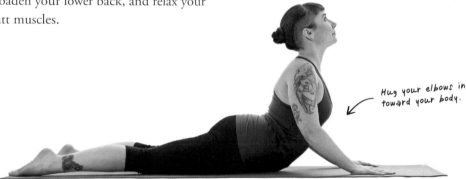

Hug your elbows in toward your body.

VARIATION: BABY COBRA

- Begin on your belly with your legs hip-width apart, palms flat on the floor next to your ribs and elbows tucked in toward your body.

- On an inhale, draw your shoulder blades down your back and pull your chest forward. Elbows stay bent and tight to your body. Gaze up and forward.

You should be able to lift your hands off the ground—most of the work is in your upper back, core, and legs.

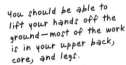

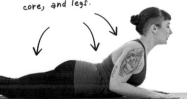

UPWARD-FACING DOG

Urdhva Mukha Svanasana

- Begin on your belly with your legs hip-width apart, your palms flat on the floor next to your ribs, and your elbows over your wrists.

- Press into your toes and engage your legs, rotate your inner thighs inward to broaden your lower back, and relax your butt muscles.

- On an inhale, press into your palms to lift your entire body from the ground, keeping the tops of your feet and your palms firmly planted to the ground.

- Allow your hips and pelvis to drop, but keep your legs straight. Lift your chest, roll your shoulders back, and pump your heart through your arms. Keep your arms straight and distribute your weight evenly across your hands. Gaze up and forward.

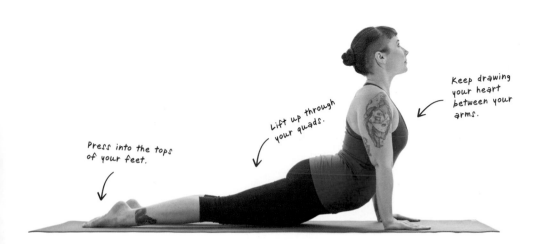

Keep drawing your heart between your arms.

Lift up through your quads.

Press into the tops of your feet.

LOCUST
Salabhasana

- Lie on your belly with your arms flat alongside you, palms down or up (depends on your mood, right?).

- Press all your toes into the ground to activate your legs, and roll your inner thighs together. Try to keep your booty relaxed.

- On an inhale, engage your core and press your pelvis and abs into the ground to draw up your chest and legs. Ultimately, you want to get your chest and legs to the same height, but don't obsess over it.

- Flex through your toes and roll your shoulders back to help your heart pump forward.

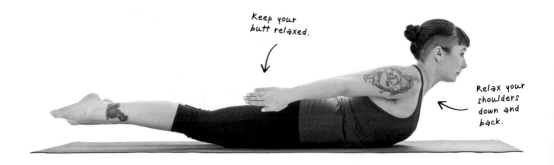

Keep your butt relaxed.

Relax your shoulders down and back.

BOW POSE
Dhanurasana

Optional Props: 1–2 straps

- Start out on your belly, stretch your arms back, bend your knees, and grab the outer edges of your feet or ankles.

- Keep your thumbs down. This foot-grab action might not happen immediately. Be patient, and grab a strap or two to hook your feet if necessary. Or just reach energetically in the direction of your feet.

- If you've got the grip, keep your legs hip-width apart and press your shins back to pump your heart forward.

- Keep shooting your thighs upward and pressing your abs and pelvis into the ground. Look forward if you want, or look up if you're feeling fearless.

As your spine becomes more flexible, as your shoulders open up, as your quads and hamstrings become more supple, and as your lower back relaxes, you will eventually be able to reach the sides of your feet.

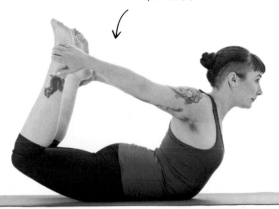

CAMEL POSE

Ustrasana

MODIFIED

- Come to kneel on the floor with your knees hip-width apart. Curl your toes under. Bring your hands to your lower back, fingers pointing down.

- With your pelvis in line with your knees, let your tailbone shoot down and engage your core in order to lift your lower belly.

- Lean back while rolling your shoulders back, hugging your elbows in toward each other, and curling your chest up and open.

- Relax your head and let your throat open up. If you'd like, release your arms and reach back for your heels. Take a few breaths and relax into the pose. Take your time coming out of the pose, and let your head come up last.

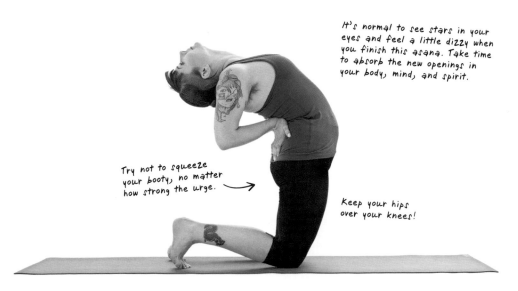

It's normal to see stars in your eyes and feel a little dizzy when you finish this asana. Take time to absorb the new openings in your body, mind, and spirit.

Try not to squeeze your booty, no matter how strong the urge. →

Keep your hips over your knees!

UNMODIFIED

- Kneel on the floor with your knees hip-width apart. Bring your hands to your lower back, fingers pointing down.

- Relax the tops of your feet flat on the ground. With your pelvis in line with your knees, let your tailbone shoot down and maintain a lifted lower belly.

- Lean back while rolling your shoulders back, hugging your elbows in, and curling your chest up and open. If you want, bring your palms to press at your heart's center. When you're ready, release your arms and reach back for your heels.

- Relax your head and let your throat open up. Take a few breaths and relax into the pose. You might feel a wave of nausea, but it usually passes as quickly as it comes. Take your time coming out of the pose, and let your head come up last.

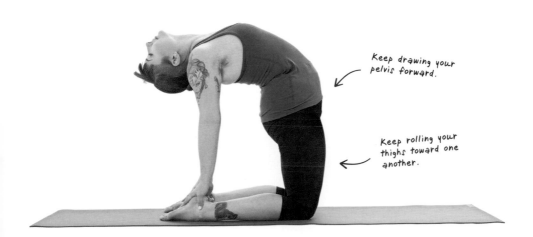

Keep drawing your pelvis forward.

Keep rolling your thighs toward one another.

BRIDGE

Setu Bandha Sarvangasana

UNSUPPORTED

- Lie on your back with your knees pointing to the sky and your feet flat on the ground, hip-width apart.

- Begin to lift your hips off the floor. Interlace your fingers behind your lower back or let your palms rest flat on the ground.

- Roll your shoulders under your chest and press evenly through all four corners of your feet to keep lifting your hips up to the height of your knees.

- Keep moving your chin away from your chest and keep your booty soft. Roll your thighs inward and down. Keep your knees rolling in, and try to keep your knees in line with your heels. Stay for a few breaths and gently lower back down.

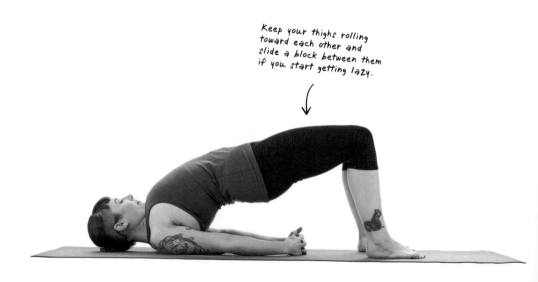

Keep your thighs rolling toward each other and slide a block between them if you start getting lazy.

SUPPORTED

Prop: 1 block

- Lie on your back with your knees pointing to the sky and your feet flat on the ground, hip-width apart.

- Begin to lift your hips off the floor. Slide a block at the tall or medium level under your sacrum and relax your hips.

- Roll your shoulders under your chest and press evenly through all four corners of your feet to keep lifting your hips up to the height of your knees. Interlace your fingers behind your lower back or let your palms rest flat on the ground.

- Keep moving your chin away from your chest and keep your booty soft. Roll your thighs inward and down. Keep your knees rolling in, and try to keep your knees in line with your heels. Stay for a few breaths and gently lower back down.

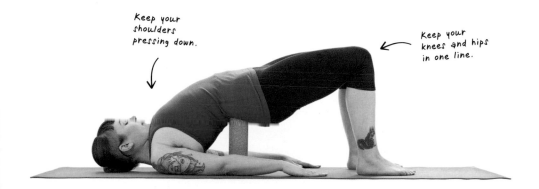

Keep your shoulders pressing down.

Keep your knees and hips in one line.

RESTORE
CHILD'S POSE
Balasana

SUPPORTED AND UNSUPPORTED

Optional Props: 1-2 blankets

- Sit on your heels and draw your knees hip-width apart (or more—I won't tell anyone).

- If you want, slide a folded blanket between your knees and the floor or roll up a blanket and slide it between your knees and thighs. Get fucking cozy.

- Fold your torso over your legs and rest your forehead on the ground and either extend your arms in front of you or let them rest next to your hips with palms up. It's cool if your booty comes up in the air a little. Release all tension in your shoulders, neck, and head, and close your eyes.

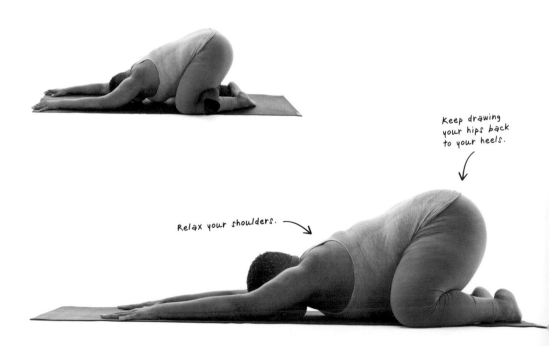

Keep drawing your hips back to your heels.

Relax your shoulders.

SEATED FORWARD BEND
Paschimottanasana

SUPPORTED AND UNSUPPORTED

Optional Props: 1 blanket, 1 strap

- Sit on your booty with your legs extended in front of you.

- Move your booty flesh from the area around your sitting bones so you can sit up nice and tall. If you want, slide a folded blanket under your sitting bones.

- Root into your hips and lean forward to catch the outer edges of your feet, working toward clasping your right wrist with the opposite hand.

- Continue to root into your hips. Inhale your heart forward and exhale to lengthen your torso forward over your legs. If your legs are tight, use a strap to catch the outer edges of your feet.

- Release tension in your neck and shoulders. Keep a bend in your knees if necessary. Actively press your thighs to the ground and flex your feet. Take several breaths, then gently roll up to seated.

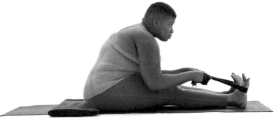

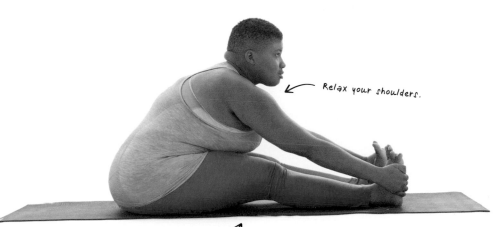

Relax your shoulders.

Keep a microbend in your knees if necessary.

BOUND ANGLE POSE
Baddha Konasana

UNSUPPORTED

- Sit on your booty, bend your knees, and bring the soles of your feet to touch with the heels tucked close to your pelvis.

- Grab hold of your feet, press your elbows into your inner thighs, and draw your head to the floor and your belly to your feet. Try not to round your spine as you fold forward. Use your elbows as anchor weights for your legs, stay for several breaths, then gently roll yourself back up.

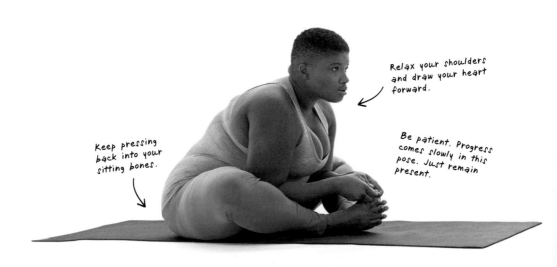

Relax your shoulders and draw your heart forward.

Keep pressing back into your sitting bones.

Be patient. Progress comes slowly in this pose. Just remain present.

SUPPORTED

Props: 1 blanket and 2 blocks

- Fold up a blanket and slide it under your booty to help yourself sit up tall. Bend your knees and bring the soles of your feet together with the heels tucked close to your pelvis.

- Take your blocks and slide one under each knee/thigh region for additional support.

- Grab hold of your feet, press your elbows into your inner thighs, and draw your head to the floor and your belly to your feet. Try not to round your spine as you fold forward. Use your elbows as anchor weights for your legs, stay for several breaths, then gently roll yourself back up.

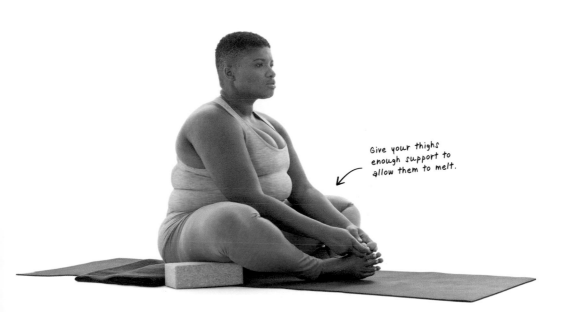

Give your thighs enough support to allow them to melt.

RECLINED BOUND ANGLE POSE

Supta Baddha Konasana

UNSUPPORTED

- Start on your back with the soles of your feet together. Snuggle your heels close to your groin.

- Take up space with your arms and let your palms face up. Relax your arms. Draw your shoulder blades down your back and let your chest lift ever so slightly. Stay here for several breaths.

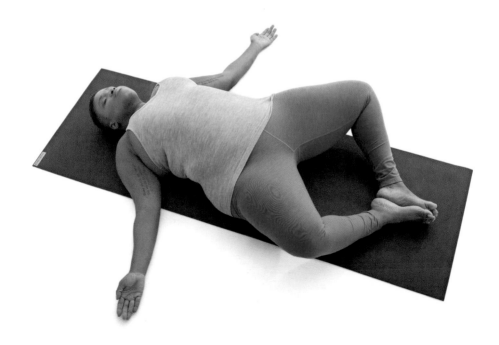

SUPPORTED

Prop: 1 bolster, 1 blanket, and 2-4 blocks

- Start on your back with the soles of your feet together. Slide a bolster mounted with the blocks under your spine lengthwise. You can also use blocks under your thighs.

- Snuggle your heels close to your groin and relax your arms on either side. Take up space with your arms and let your palms face up. Draw your shoulder blades down your back and let your chest lift ever so slightly. Stay here for several breaths.

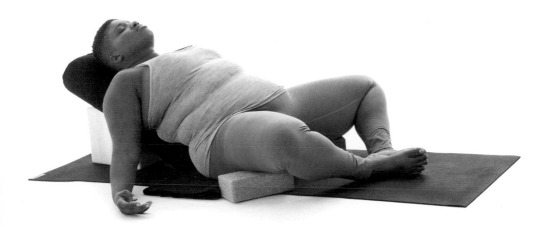

CORPSE POSE

Savasana

UNSUPPORTED

- Lie on your back. You can also feel free to collapse, fall, or whatever else your body needs to do. This pose is best served after a demanding practice, so no dignity required.

- Let your legs and arms open up, with the palms facing up. Slide your shoulder blades down your back and lift your chest ever so slightly.

- Work toward releasing all tension in your body. Close your eyes, and consider draping a piece of fabric across them to block out daylight.

- Steady your breath, let your mind relax, and simply rest.

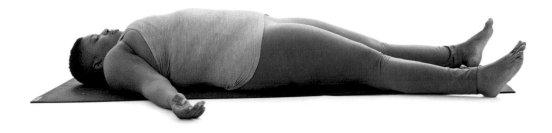

SUPPORTED

Props: whatever you want

- Lie on your back.

- Let your legs and arms open up, with the palms facing up. Slide your shoulder blades down your back and lift your chest ever so slightly.

- Work toward releasing all tension in your body. Close your eyes, and consider draping a piece of fabric across them to block out daylight. I like to slide a bolster under my spine lengthwise, or maybe under my knees widthwise. Some like to drape a blanket across their body or use the blanket as a rolled-up ankle brace. Use whatever props you want, but get very cozy.

- Steady your breath, let your mind relax, and simply rest.

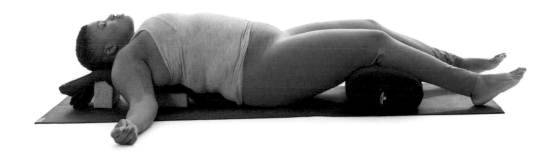

QUESTIONS ASKED BY (LITERALLY) EVERY BEGINNER YOGA STUDENT

WHY IS DOWNWARD-FACING DOG SO DIFFICULT?

I can't tell you how many times I've been asked this question, and it's because Downward-Facing Dog (page 80) is difficult for nearly all new yoga practitioners. Often, this is because many people hold all the weight in their wrists, one of our most tender bodily regions. Bearing too much weight into the wrist is painful and can cause long-term damage, including carpal tunnel and arthritis. The key to holding your Downward-Facing Dogs without wanting to kill yourself and your yoga instructor? CLAW THE MAT. Plug into your fingertips and knuckles when you step into the pose—this will create a kind of suction cup in the palm of your hand that will protect your wrist and be *much* more comfortable overall. This grip will allow you to balance the weight of your body between both your top *and* bottom halves, as opposed to bearing the full weight of your body into one joint. Also, if the pose becomes too difficult (trust me, it happens to everyone), drop down to your knees in Modified High Plank (page 95) and practice "clawing the mat"—make a suction cup in your palms and strengthen through your full arm and shoulder while on your knees—then, when you're feeling confident, lift your knees and return to Downward-Facing Dog. Repetition is the key—the only way to really feel change and growth with any asana (especially Downward-Facing Dog) is to keep going, even when the going gets rough.

OKAY, BUT WHAT IF MY BODY CAN'T MAKE ANY OF THESE SHAPES AT ALL?

There are a million reasons why you might think your body is specifically ill-equipped to practice yoga asana. Maybe you are coming to yoga immediately after having a baby or after suffering a major injury. Maybe you think that I'm too "skinny fat" to understand the struggles of a *real* fat person. The fact of the matter is that yoga is for everyone, regardless of what's going on in your personal life saga.

Some of the most amazing yoga success stories have sprung from the practices of people who faced incredible odds. For example, I remember watching a YouTube video about an army vet who broke both his legs while serving as a paratrooper. Over the course of two years, he went from being completely immobile to sprinting down the street, and he attributed his success to yoga. Also, one of my most influential yoga instructors practiced the extremely rigorous and demanding Bikram asana sequence essentially up until her baby's due date, with no negative repercussions. Stephanie Keach, another influential teacher of mine, didn't even *start* practicing yoga until after suffering a serious back injury that had left her completely bedridden. Yoga asana healed her body when it was at its weakest.

If your body is injured, it's most important to accept that your yoga poses may not look like everyone else's. That's okay. Just adapt the poses to your current state of being. If you can't move your legs, work on the asana shapes that occur in the top region of your body instead. If you have a broken arm, work on your standing poses. And always have props on hand to cushion your sensitive body parts, such as blankets to slide under tender knees or blocks to support sensitive wrists and replaced hip joints. Set your own pace and be okay with moving slower than other people in the room.

You may notice that I didn't mention any miraculous stories of fat people "overcoming miraculous odds" in order to practice yoga. That's because being fat isn't an injury or an impediment—fatness merely needs to be accommodated. If you're fat and practicing yoga, make space for your extra flesh. Spread your knees and thighs farther apart in poses like Child's Pose (page 124) to accommodate your body or keep your large breasts from falling in your face by tightening a yoga strap across the top region of your chest. But the most important thing is to stop seeing your fat body as an injury—in that situation, the only injured body part is your mind.

I DON'T HAVE A LOT OF STRENGTH IN MY ARMS AND LEGS, AND EVERY KIND OF EXERCISE (YOGA INCLUDED) IS EXTREMELY HARD FOR ME. WHAT SHOULD I DO?

Anyone who exhibits extreme strength, flexibility, or agility will tell you that those abilities didn't come easily. Strength is garnered over time, and it is usually hard won. Just because you don't feel strong today doesn't mean you won't feel strong after a few months of vigorous yoga classes. It's natural for the yoga to be hard in the beginning—I mean, YOU'VE NEVER DONE IT BEFORE. But you owe it to yourself to actually give it an honest try, because when you give yourself a chance on your yoga mat, you give yourself a chance in other parts of your life.

HOW DO I KNOW WHEN I'M ADVANCED ENOUGH FOR A NONBEGINNER YOGA CLASS?

This is the thing about yoga—we're all always beginners. Every time you come to your mat, you should arrive brimming with childlike enthusiasm and optimism, fully willing to learn something new and step out into uncharted territory. That being said, there are definitely classes that might kick your ass harder than others. But that doesn't mean you shouldn't be willing to give them a shot. After all, won't there always be a harder version of *something* in our lives? There are a million opportunities to shortchange yourself on a daily basis; don't let it happen with your yoga practice. In short, with the exception of classes that specifically indicate the need for advanced skills, I'd say GO FOR IT!

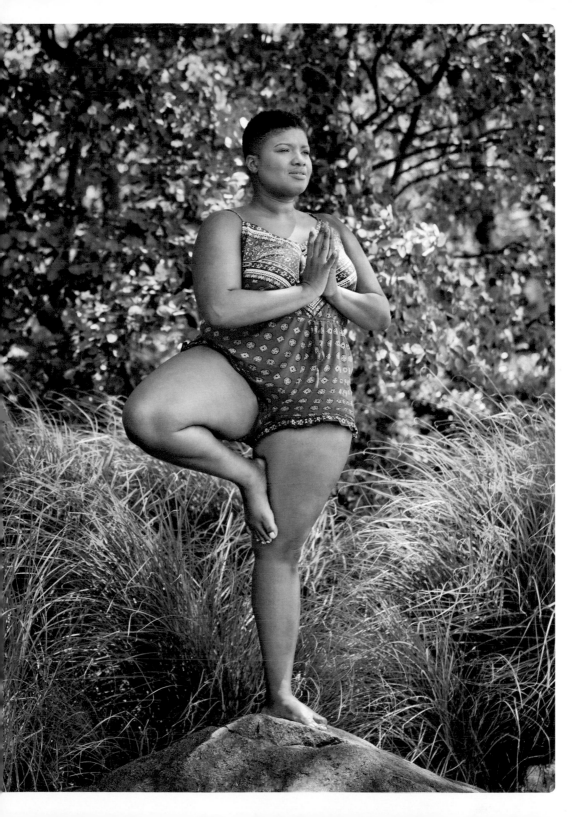

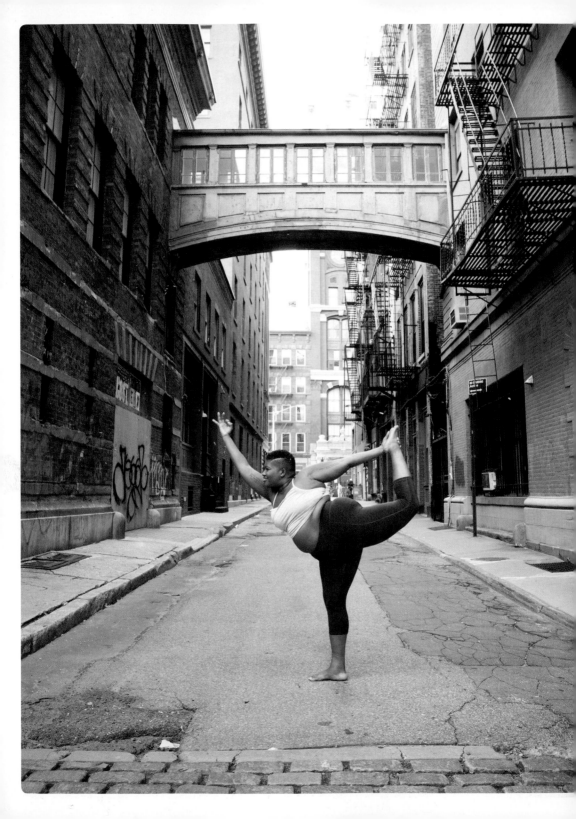

PART 4

Okay, But How Can I Do This on My Own?

HOW I LEARNED MY ASANA ABCS

I doubt I would have felt such an insuppressible urge to get on my mat day after day had it not been for the ridiculous antics of my life *off* the mat. I am grateful for all of my life experiences, even the nasty ones. Were it not for universal confrontations with death, heartache, relationship turmoil, infidelity, and (seriously) so much more, it's possible my yoga practice wouldn't exist at all. And I don't want to hide my uglier moments. I want to embrace them. Those ugly moments are the real reason I've been able to learn my asana ABCs. And I think that if you too embrace your uglier moments, you'll be able to learn *your* asana ABCs as well. I genuinely believe that openhearted honesty about the complexities of our lives is the key to spreading Patanjali's eight-limbed path into a whole new generation of practitioners.

In my asana practice, as in life, I've tripped, fallen, busted my ass, and had to manually scrape myself off the pavement. And as a result, my yoga practice is now a fertile and fulfilling foundation of my life. Creative, dynamic sequencing really made the difference in my understanding of asana, and I owe much of my asana knowledge to a regular practice of the sequences sprinkled throughout this section. I've designed the sequencing suggestions here as the kindling for your vinyasa-style yoga practice. Mix and match the sequences into the perfect practice for your day.

BRING IT ON, BITCH

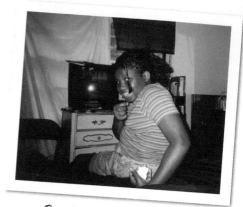

The original Awkward Black Girl

By the time middle school rolled around, I was fat, awkward, and SO not cool. "Cool" for tweenage Jessamyn meant size 4 jeans from Abercrombie & Fitch, an extensive Beanie Baby collection, and a trendy knapsack chock-full of Bonne Bell Lip Smackers and multicolored glitter gel pens. It did *not*, in any way, shape, or form, mean size 12 jeans from Walmart, guffaws of parental laughter in response to requests for Beanie Babies, and dollar-store versions of every other trinkety accessory under the sun. My middle school was smack dab in the middle of Southern suburbia, and my lower-middle-class chubby black weirdness didn't have a chance in hell of achieving the kind of popularity and utter coolness that seemed to be the norm for my upper-middle-class classmates. Nevertheless, becoming "cool" was the primary extracurricular of my middle school years. And at Jamestown Middle School, during the peak of MTV-heralded beauty ideals, cheerleaders were the absolute epitome of cool.

I blame my weird cheerleading obsession on the quintessential high school motion picture *Bring It On*. If you've never seen it, I would highly recommend that you watch it ASAP. *Bring It On* was a teenybopper classic of the early 2000s and, if you know a femme who was between the ages of eleven and fourteen at the dawn of the new millennium, there's a good chance she's an undercover fan of this film. The movie's premise pits two sassy rival team captains against each other in one epic battle of cheerleading badassery. It glorified cheerleading culture—the catty attitudes, the matching outfits and makeup, the razor-sharp, precise back handsprings, and the misogynistic and racially problematic choreographed dances. The camaraderie and shared stereotypical beauty of all the characters was intoxicating and infectious. I idolized the film's heroines and became convinced that there was a bubbly, coordinated, flexible cheerleader buried deep within my chubby, inflexible, uncoordinated frame.

Becoming "cool" was the primary extracurricular of my middle school years.

To be clear, this wasn't my first foray into graceful movement. After a pre–grade school introduction to the cinematic magic of *The Red Shoes*, I developed an early and rabid fetish for the dancer lifestyle. I was always particularly fond of ballet culture—the tights, leotards, toe shoes, and classical music always struck me as incredibly glamorous. While an elementary school student, I took ballet, tap, and jazz classes that I absolutely adored. I dreamed of magically waking from a Sleeping Beauty–esque rest to have acquired the willowy stature of a dancer, and to move gracefully across a spotlit stage while barely grazing the floor with my pale pink toe shoes.

Instead, what my childhood dance classes showcased was an embarrassingly obvious lack of natural flexibility and coordination, skills typically found in both professional dancers *and* cheerleaders. Although my flexibility and coordination left much to the imagination, I still considered myself a reasonably competent dancer, and I reasoned that I could probably gradually develop the other typical cheerleader skills. After all, I'd seen photos of curvy-bodied cheerleaders, and there was usually at least one girl on my middle school squad who rocked a plus-size cheer uniform.

But I could never do any of the requisite cheerleader Cirque du Soleil–style party tricks. The best cheerleaders, even the fat ones, were always popping up into air splits, dropping cartwheels left and right, and back handspringing for days on end. It probably goes without saying that

I was completely incapable of doing any of that shit. However, thanks to years of family-funded artistic expression, I'd been blessed with the kind of inflated ego that can only come as the result of tireless parental emotional coddling. Therefore, I was pretty well convinced that with a little practice, self-motivation, and a good seamstress I could find my way into a plus-size cheer uniform of my very own.

Unfortunately, the Jamestown Middle School cheerleading team did not agree with my assessment. I'm being kind when I say that I absolutely sucked and blew my tryout. The standard pre-practice jogging, a staple of every cheerleading practice from here to Timbuktu, struck me as a form of medieval torture. Even though I had danced across many a stage and even tried my hand at kid-friendly gymnastics and tae kwon do, I was not a childhood athletic prodigy, and traditional running has been my nemesis from day 1. But I huffed and puffed my way through the cheerleading tryout warm-ups, not unlike the rhinoceros who lags in the jungle animal stampede at the end of *Jumanji*. By the time I found my way to the finish line of the cheerleading running circuits, I was probably already disqualified from the team's most JV roster. I mean, what difference did my lackluster dancing skills make when I could barely finish the fucking WARM-UP exercises?

> *I felt supremely ugly and excluded, and this became the furnace fuel for a rapidly blooming bottomless pit of self-disgust.*

And so I shuffle-ball-changed my fat ass away from cheerleading caviar dreams and I saddled on an additional load of body discomfort. Even though my logical mind understood that being able to complete basic warm-up exercises was the most essential aspect of any *Bring It On*–worthy cheer success story, my illogical emotions and ego were completely unwilling to get on the right page. I felt supremely ugly and excluded, and this became the furnace fuel for a rapidly blooming bottomless pit of self-disgust.

LESSONS LEARNED

Sun salutations make it better. When you find yourself settling into a pit of self-hate and anger, it's time to get your ass up and do some sun salutations. If you're feeling down about yourself, do a sun salutation. If you need a little pick-me-up, do a sun salutation. Think of it as yogic cocaine—or yogic caffeine, if that makes you more comfortable.

Sun salutations are a popular sequence of asana that are usually performed as a stand-alone sequence or as the beginning to a longer yoga flow sequence. They are designed to invite prana, that delicious vital life source, into every part of your body—think of it as insulation against internal negativity.

Each pose in the sequence invites warmth and energy into a different part of your body, reminding it of the strength and power of the sun. Some people like to practice sun salutes first thing in the morning. Others like to sleep in, go to work late, get pissed off halfway through the day, and do three sun salutes in a row for focus and energy. You don't even have to do them from a standing position: You can keep your ass seated in a chair and just do the arm movements and forward-folding shapes. It doesn't matter how you slice it—sun salutes will wake up your life and allow your heart to smile wide open to the universe.

I like to start my home asana practice with three rounds of Sun Salutation A. The number three is a sacred number in yoga, and it represents a sense of balance in life. Each round of Sun Salutation A progressively wakes up my body and makes me feel more relaxed and open to the physical vigor of any asana to come.

Whereas Sun Salutation A is a pretty realistic interpretation of a human *literally* saluting the sun, Sun Salutation B is WAY more intense—kind of like having the sun shine directly out of your ass at a million watts per minute. By adding a couple of extra poses and some vigorous movement, the internal *tapas* (heat) is kicked up ten million notches for a much more physically intense experience. You will get sweaty and your body will tremble like a motherfucker. That's good. Invite it in.

SUN SALUTATION

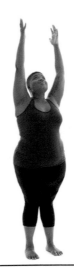

Root into
the ground.

1. MOUNTAIN POSE (PAGE 74)

2. UPWARD SALUTE (PAGE 75)

Round through
upper back.

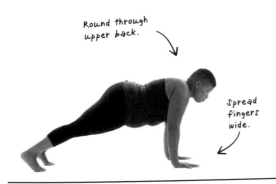

Spread
fingers
wide.

Grip into
the ground.

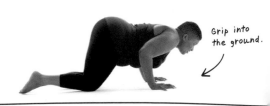

5. HIGH PLANK (PAGE 94)

**6. MODIFIED FOUR-LIMBED
STAFF POSE (PAGE 96)**

A rich ujjayi breath is recommended for this type of movement. (See page 65.)

Lengthen through your spine.

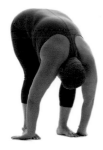

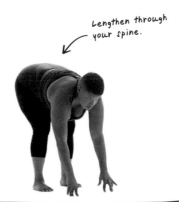

3. STANDING FORWARD FOLD (PAGE 76)

4. STANDING HALF FORWARD FOLD (PAGE 78)

Lift up hips and back.

Keep pelvis heavy.

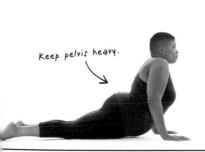

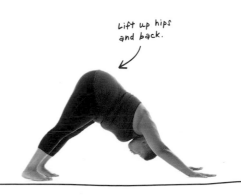

7. COBRA (PAGE 116) OR UPWARD-FACING DOG (PAGE 117)

8. DOWNWARD-FACING DOG (PAGE 80)

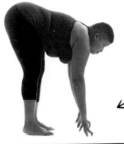

Walk or hop your feet to your hands.

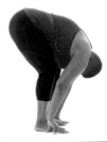

9. STANDING HALF FORWARD FOLD (PAGE 78)

10. STANDING FORWARD FOLD (PAGE 76)

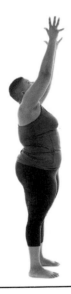

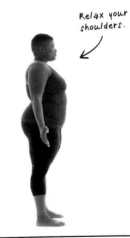

Relax your shoulders.

11. UPWARD SALUTE (PAGE 75)

12. MOUNTAIN POSE (PAGE 74)

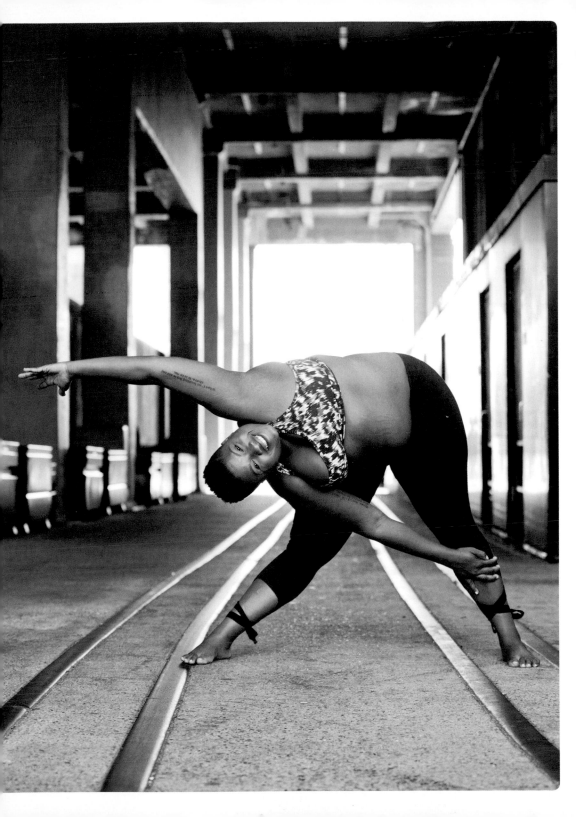

SUN SALUTATION

Following a few rounds of Sun Salutation A, I like to roll through two rounds of Sun Salutation B. Sometimes, if my body is really feeling it, I'll add a third round—sometimes the energy just feels too good to stop.

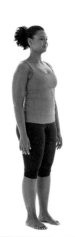

1. MOUNTAIN POSE (PAGE 74)

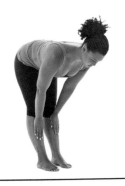

5. STANDING HALF FORWARD FOLD (PAGE 78)

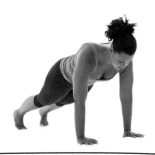

6. HIGH PLANK (PAGE 94)

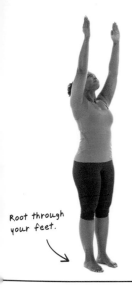

Root through
your feet.

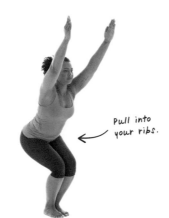

Pull into
your ribs.

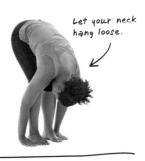

Let your neck
hang loose.

2. UPWARD SALUTE (PAGE 75)

3. CHAIR POSE (PAGE 82)

4. STANDING FORWARD FOLD (PAGE 76)

Hug your elbows
to your sides.

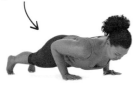

Lift your pelvis.

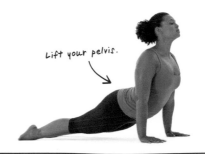

7. FOUR-LIMBED STAFF POSE (PAGE 96)

8. COBRA (PAGE 116) OR UPWARD-FACING DOG (PAGE 117)

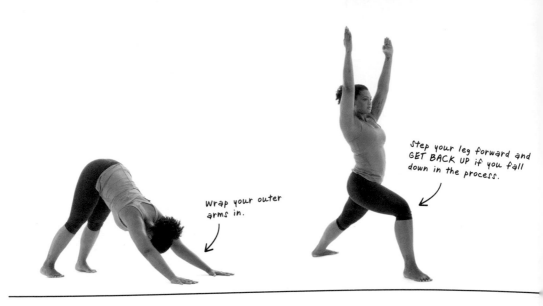

Wrap your outer arms in.

Step your leg forward and GET BACK UP if you fall down in the process.

9. DOWNWARD-FACING DOG (PAGE 80)

10. WARRIOR 1 (PAGE 83)

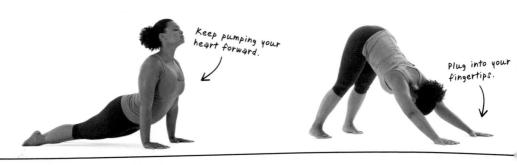

Keep pumping your heart forward.

Plug into your fingertips.

13. COBRA POSE (PAGE 116) OR UPWARD-FACING DOG (PAGE 117)

14. DOWNWARD-FACING DOG (PAGE 80)

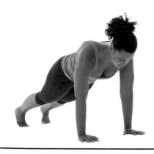

11. HIGH PLANK (PAGE 94)

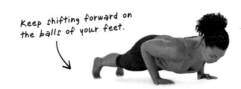

Keep shifting forward on the balls of your feet.

12. FOUR-LIMBED STAFF (PAGE 96)

15–19: Repeat steps 10 to 14, beginning on your alternate leg.

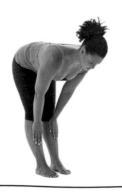

20. STANDING HALF FORWARD FOLD (PAGE 78)

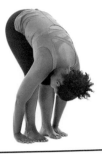

21. STANDING FORWARD FOLD (PAGE 76)

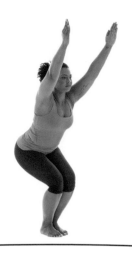

22. CHAIR POSE (PAGE 82)

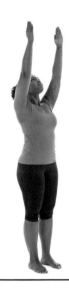

23. UPWARD SALUTE (PAGE 75)

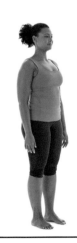

24. MOUNTAIN POSE (PAGE 74)

THE OREO

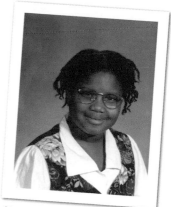

Pioneering the Harry Potter look
way back in '95.

By the end of fourth grade, I'd sustained enough failed puppy love crushes on my Jonathan Taylor Thomas–inspired male classmates to realize I didn't really fit into the traditional definition of pretty. Thanks to my subscriptions to *Teen* and *Seventeen* (which I read religiously and held in the absolute highest esteem), I was very familiar with society's agreed-upon vision of beauty. And, as much as it pained me to admit it, I knew for sure that the accepted image didn't have jack shit to do with me.

However, I grew up the daughter/granddaughter/niece of a long and dignified lineage of proud, black, curvy women. Just like my magazine subscriptions, I held their judgments in high regard. I knew my mother, my aunts, and my grandmothers to be the absolute epitome and essence of beauty, and I took comfort in the fact that even if I didn't look like Katie Holmes on *Dawson's Creek*, at least I looked sort of like the powerful women who were present in my daily life. It wasn't much to stand on, but this understanding of beauty kept me mostly afloat through my elementary school years.

When I was in third grade, as a way to punctuate our natural Afro-American beauty, my mother twisted both of our hair into locs. For Tangela, this decision was an amazing way for us to reclaim our strong black heritage while deflecting the beauty ideals that a white-centric society viciously thrusts upon the lives of black women.

To say I was "less interested" in reclaiming our heritage would be a gross understatement. My elementary school was a pretty even mix of peachy-hued white girls with strawberry blond ponytails and chocolate-caramel-coated black girls with bone-straight permed bobs. Natural hairstyles were very much *not* the norm. I didn't know anyone else outside of my family who had dreadlocked hair. And frankly, I didn't give a single fuck about anything that didn't involve my transformation into a 1990s sitcom star.

Today, as she nears her fifty-fifth birthday, Tangela's twisted hair still grows shiny, long, and magnificent. My mom's locs carry the history of her own personal struggles, especially the period when she was ill. As she triumphed over her illness, her locs grew even longer and more luscious. *My* hair, however—well, it didn't have the same fate.

I was convinced that my hair made me stick out like a sore thumb even more than I already did. It wasn't enough that I was already the resident "fat girl" of my class. I'd made the mistake of selecting Harry Potter–ish round, tortoise-rimmed glasses at my optometrist's office the summer before third grade, and the two light brown rings propped on my cherubic cheeks only seemed to accentuate my resemblance to an oven-baked Pillsbury Doughboy. And none of my clothes ever fit quite right. My mother was the queen of frugality, and that extended all the way to the Stanley family wardrobe. My clothing collection was a mélange of gently worn hand-me-downs from my older cousins and Walmart clearance rack numbers. By the time I hit fourth grade, I felt that I'd fully transitioned into my new identity as the Crispy Brown Pillsbury Doughgirl, and my locs only made things worse.

I guess it didn't really help that the kids already made fun of me for another reason. They even used a really clever nickname: "Oreo."

For many of you, an Oreo might be a popular chocolate sandwich cookie, one that evokes really comforting memories. If someone came up

I didn't give a single fuck about anything that didn't involve my transformation into a 1990s sitcom star.

behind you on the playground and shouted, "OREO!" you might get really excited. Because, well . . . cookies. But when I was a kid and someone came up behind me and shouted "OREO!" they probably were not talking about fucking cookies.

The black-and-white color combo of those infamous cookies inspired one of the most popular insults for black kids who, like me, enjoyed doing "white people shit," such as reading Baby-Sitters Club books, pretending to be Gwen Stefani in the "Just a Girl" music video, memorizing the entirety of Jewel's *Pieces of You*, and other things that were generally deemed to be "not black enough." Sometimes it was enough to simply have a tone of voice that suggested we obviously frequented a lot of white-kid slumber parties.

"Oreos": Black on the outside, white on the inside.

"Oreos": Black on the outside, white on the inside.

I have to say that I was at a disadvantage in this department. I mean, I *did* seem to know a lot of white people. For one thing, my strict Baháʼí upbringing meant that my family mixed in very diverse circles. The Baháʼí Faith emphasizes the importance of a new world order in which all human beings are equal to each other, no matter race or gender. As a result, the supporting characters of my childhood closely resemble a yuppie version of the original Broadway cast of *Hair*. People of all shades and persuasions came into and out of my life, and I spent much of my early childhood fairly unaware that my skin color was different than that of *anyone*, let alone that of my white friends.

As a result, being called an "Oreo" by both my white *and* black classmates was a deafening blow. I mean, the black kids thought I was trying to be white. The white kids, well . . . the white kids probably didn't give a fuck. They probably just said it because they heard other kids saying it and, let's face it, kids can just be straight-up assholes.

I, on the other hand, gave many fucks. I gave many a fuck, indeed. I felt as though I was being cast aside by all of my peers, and all because I was in an Ann M. Martin fan club and had "weird" hair. And so, along with my Lisa Frank holographic Trapper Keeper, I hauled around my hair-related

> I was being cast aside by all of my peers, and all because I was in an Ann M. Martin fan club and had "weird" hair.

self-hate for the rest of my elementary school years.

Over time, however, it became very apparent that I wasn't the only one who didn't like my hair. In fact, some of my mom's very close friends didn't think locked hair was an appropriate look for a young girl. I mean, god forbid anyone think she was the daughter of negligent, pot-smoking Rastafarians, right?[14] Nowadays, you can easily find images of natural black hair, but in the mid-1990s it was extremely common for black women to throw shade on Afrocentric natural hairstyles. "Black Beauty" of the 1990s exhibited very little variation. Our options were basically either Naomi Campbell's *My Little Pony*–inspired white-girl weaves, Nia Long's no-frills but heavily relaxed gamine cut, or Janet Jackson's *Poetic Justice* box braids. Natural hair icons, or even just a couple of famous faces with locked hair or afros, were few and far between.

So, unbeknownst to my mother, while she was being diagnosed with congestive heart failure and, you know, trying *not* to die on an operating table, one of her best friends cut off all my dreadlocks, soaked my scalp with hair relaxer to tame my natural curls, and wove my hair into crochet braids for the first time.

In retrospect, I should've swatted away the hands that were so ready to free me of my natural hairstyle. But I was ten years old and tired of being the ugly fat girl. I knew it would upset and confuse my mother, but I was hungry for acceptance by my peers—no matter the cost.

(It probably goes without saying that my mother nearly sustained a heart attack when she saw my new hairstyle and had to be physically restrained from throttling the main person involved in cutting my hair. In the end, Tangela basically cut everyone involved in my new 'do out of our lives.)

---

14 This is the part where I acknowledge that even black people can be racist against other black people. This is a very real thing, y'all.

I didn't know it at the time, but the decision to cut off my natural locs and braid my hair was an emotionally arresting experience. After that point, I became scared to show my natural hair to people. I concealed a crucial aspect of my identity from the outside world and, in effect, from myself. I see now that renouncing my natural hair was the start of a very confusing cycle of identity problems with my Afro-American heritage, which continued into my early adulthood. In a myriad ways, the repression of my natural hair sparked a repression of my identity as a powerful black woman, causing untold damage to my emotional and spiritual strength. I would continue to wear my naturally kinky hair in some sort of braided style for the next thirteen years.

LESSON LEARNED

There's a part of me that wishes I could go back in time Marty McFly–style and tell Kid Jessamyn that it's okay to be different from everyone else. That it's fine to be weird. That you don't have to look like everyone else. That even if your hairstyle is different from all the other little girls', you're still a cool person. But it's useless to wish those things. I needed to have those experiences, and I needed to feel that pain. One way or another, I had to start the process of ignoring the concerns of other people.

As a beginner yoga student, it's totally normal to walk into a yoga studio and feel like you're standing on the outskirts of a secret little clique— an embarrassed outcast with nowhere to hide. And as the only chubby black person in my early yoga classes, I definitely had a few "Oreo" flashbacks.

I don't really believe in "yoga for beginners"—I think most people are capable of practicing most styles of yoga, provided they are taught in "all levels" classes where the instructor offers options for both advanced practitioners and novices. However, I'm willing to accept many new students might want a flow that provides a stepping stone before they take off the training wheels.

I WANT TO GET

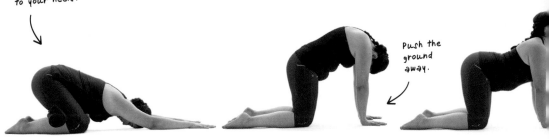

Keep shifting your hips back to your heels.

Push the ground away.

1. CHILD'S POSE (SUPPORTED, PAGE 124)

2. CAT/COW POSE (PAGE 114)

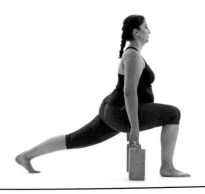

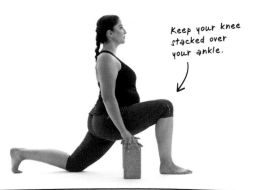

Keep your knee stacked over your ankle.

5. HIGH LUNGE POSE (SUPPORTED, PAGE 105)

6. LOW LUNGE POSE (SUPPORTED, PAGE 106)

STARTED

Before doing this flow, you can start with a few rounds of Sun Salutation A (page 144) or Sun Salutation B (page 148), or you can simply start by establishing a strong, robust ujjayi breath (page 65).

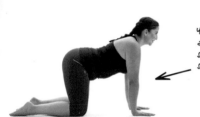

Your shoulders and wrists should be stacked.

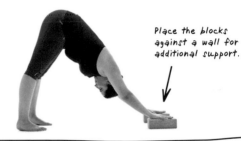

Place the blocks against a wall for additional support.

3. HIGH PLANK (MODIFIED, PAGE 95)

4. DOWNWARD-FACING DOG (SUPPORTED, PAGE 81)

9–14 Repeat sequence on alternate leg.

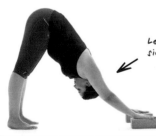

Lengthen through the sides of your body.

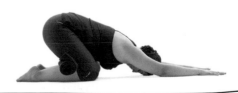

7. DOWNWARD-FACING DOG (SUPPORTED, PAGE 81)

8. CHILD'S POSE (SUPPORTED, PAGE 124)

JESSAMYN STANLEY, PRE-TEEN BEAUTY QUEEN

When I was eleven years old, I decided to enter the Miss Pre-Teen North Carolina Pageant. I promise you, I'm not joking.

I wish I could tell you why I did it. I'm sure my parents are still wondering the exact same thing. To their credit, Jesse and Tangela were against the whole pageant scheme from the jump-off, and not just because we were entirely too poor to afford all the trimmings of turn-of-the-twenty-first-century American pageantry. But I think maybe they realized that Pre-Teen Jessamyn was obviously enduring a very poor transition from kiddie-dom to pre-menstruation and had slipped into some sort of mildly embarrassing early adolescent crisis. This was presumably the same life crisis that had also led me down the confusing path of trying to live out a cheerleading movie.

If that's the case, I choose to believe they didn't want to make things any worse by suggesting I avoid potential hot shame and searing embarrassment that were both totally at stake if I entered a beauty pageant. Because I was hell-bent and determined to be a pageant queen. No lie, it probably had something to do with one of my other favorite Kirsten Dunst flicks, *Drop Dead Gorgeous*.[15] Also, I'm not ruling out that it could have been a weirdly morbid and inappropriate reaction to the murder of JonBenet

Ramsey. Honestly, it was probably in large part because I harbored serious doubts about my natural beauty and needed reassurance that I was pretty.

Anyway, for whatever the reason, I decided to enter the Miss Pre-Teen North Carolina Pageant.

On the day of our little local pageant, I was cute and had precocious, rambling Velveeta cheesy responses to every interview question. During the talent portion, I squeezed into my YMCA "Cheer America" cheerleading team uniform and performed a few highly choreographed pom-pom shakes and head bobs. I figured that though my obsession with cheerleading culture wasn't deemed worthwhile by my school's team, it could at least help me snag the hearts of local celebrity judges. I smiled at every judge like they were the apple of my eye, and I sashayed down the runway like a soon-to-be-disqualified *RuPaul's Drag Race* contestant.

> *I needed reassurance that I was pretty.*

You may be surprised to learn that I WAS THE MOTHERFUCKING FIRST RUNNER-UP. SECOND PLACE, BITCHES.

(I BET YOU DIDN'T SEE THAT COMING.[16])

I mean, at the time it seemed completely improbable, because I was well aware of my lack of traditional pretty-girl characteristics. But even I have to admit—I made a stellar local pageant girl. I was absolutely thrilled—my victory at the state level meant that I was eligible to compete at the national level. So my mom and I booked a hotel room, kissed my dad and little brother good-bye, and got our asses down to Florida for the Miss Pre-Teen America Pageant.

Or maybe it was called Miss Pre-Teen Nationals? Hmmm. I honestly can't remember. My memories of this episode are fairly vague, and I think it's because I've purposefully blocked out major chunks of the whole experience.

---

15 Damn, Kirsten really _was_ the poster girl for tweens of the early 2000s. I have no idea why I felt such a strong connection with this particular teen queen, but I'm not going to question it. Forget Winona (apparently): Kirsten Forever.

16 That's what we call a plot twist.

In preparation for the big day, my mom and I went from store to store, scouring the racks of prom dresses, bridesmaid gowns, and Quinceañera gowns for a formal pageant gown that would both hold in my back fat and not make me resemble a dark-chocolate-frosted cupcake, while simultaneously not costing a million dollars and requiring our family to seek government assistance. We eventually found a size 12 canary yellow satin gown at a bridal outlet in Burlington, North Carolina, a gown I loved to the point of donning it for every formal family event for the following two years, long after I'd outgrown the size 12 and moved firmly into the realm of US 14–16.

I distinctly recall arriving in Florida and being thrilled to check in to our hotel room at Orlando's notoriously opulent Peabody Hotel.[17] I remember being introduced to my pageant-week roommate, a multi-pageant champion from Chicago, and her mother, a woman who managed to evoke the spirit of Mama Rose but with the Diet Pepsi tartness of Peg Bundy. Those two were a true pageant dynamic duo, and I remember being blown away by their utter dedication to the art of *winning*.

The daughter, following in the footsteps of her former pageant queen mother, had been competing in large-scale pageants since she was reasonably old enough to simultaneously toddle across a stage and twirl a baton. I was in awe of her discipline and talent—her smile was always perfect, her hair even more so, and she walked down the stage as though she had been professionally trained. In fact, I'm sure she *was* professionally trained. I had nowhere near her training, but I was still pretty confident. After all, my cheerleader shoulder bobs and saccharine-sweet interview answers had gotten my sassy ass all the way from the booming motel ballroom metropolis of Greensboro, North Carolina, to Orlando, Florida. In my humble estimation, it seemed highly unlikely that I wouldn't be able to snag one of the competition's top spots.

It seemed highly unlikely that I wouldn't be able to snag one of the competition's top spots.

---

17 Because I didn't grow up with a lot of money, hotel stays have always struck me as the height of glamour.

But I didn't snag one of the top spots. I didn't even clear the first round of the eliminations. To be fair, we can't all be winners in that type of situation—I mean, there are fifty fucking states and only twenty-five top spots, so that math essentially requires that a whole bunch of tweenage girls will end the night in tears. Up until that point, the only time I'd seen that many pre-teen girls communally crying was during the final drowning sequence of *Titanic* at my local movie theater.

The pit of self-disgust was growing larger, darker, and much more depressing.

I was one of the many weeping little girls. I was mortified, to say the least—mere entry into the pageant had cost my family an inordinate amount of money, and I was horribly embarrassed to have lost in such a dramatic fashion. I cried so much and so publicly that my mother scooped me up and carried my sad ass all the way back to North Carolina in THE MIDDLE OF THE NIGHT while the pageant was still chugging along.

Looking back now, I wonder why Tangela was so insistent that we go back home immediately. Probably because she didn't want our professionally poised and coiffed mommy/daughter pageant roomies to see what a sore loser her daughter could be when faced with white-hot shame and rejection.

While I won't deny that I've definitely been known to be a Stage Five Level Sore Loser, I think it was more than embarrassment that sent me scurrying home in the middle of the night. Before the national pageant, I had never fully understood just how *not pretty* I was by society's standards. I mean, I'm going to trust that you don't live under a rock and you've at least seen snippets of a televised beauty pageant before. The obsessive, shiny, beauty product–centric world that's portrayed in pop culture? It is absolutely NOT a myth—the moms and daughters are *actually* that intense, and a lot of impressionable young girls pay the price. And even though I knew my looks weren't appreciated by my schoolmates, it was another issue entirely to realize just how much they weren't appreciated by the world at large, and on a humiliating scale like that of a national beauty pageant. The pit of self-disgust that I'd been digging since my cheerleading disaster was growing larger, darker, and much more depressing. It became the catalyst for a number of questionable future decisions as I grew increasingly incapable of accepting the beautiful identity trapped beneath my distorted expectations.

LESSON LEARNED

Looking back on my childhood, what with the random pageants, cheerleading, and whatnot, it seems pretty obvious that I was ravenous for recognition and attention. I don't really think that's a flaw—I mean, it's kind of natural for humans to desire recognition, right? However, a sense of internal strength and power can feed that same need. If we can believe in ourselves and stand strong on our own, without the support or encouragement of others, we're much less likely to fall prey to foolhardy attempts at getting attention. Use the following sequence to help give you strength and power whenever you find it difficult to harness those emotions on your own.

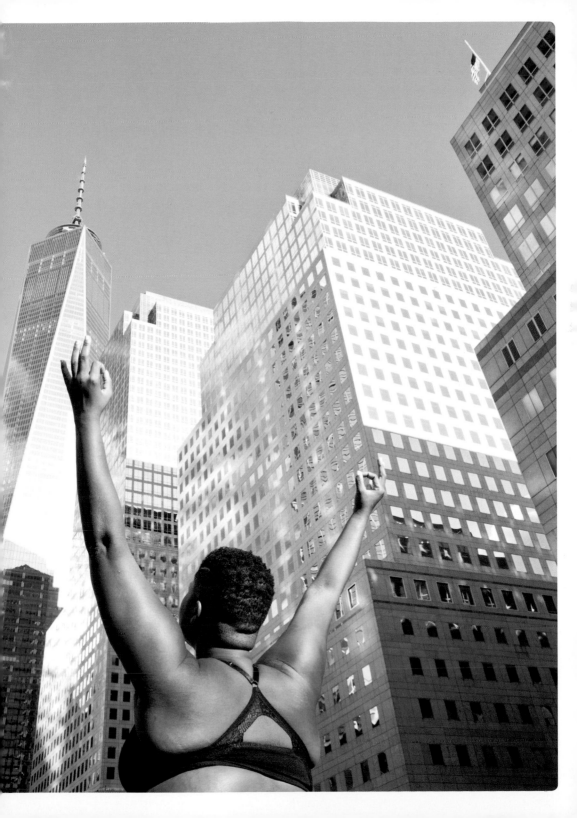

I WANT TO

Begin with three rounds of Sun Salutation A (page 144) and one or two rounds of Sun Salutation B (page 148)

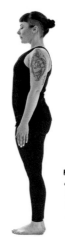

Root through all four corners of your feet, keep your hips and heels in one line, relax your shoulders.

I. MOUNTAIN POSE (PAGE 74)

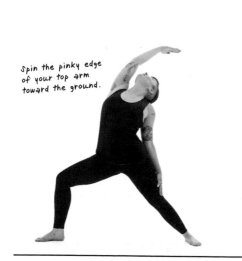

Spin the pinky edge of your top arm toward the ground.

Take a vinyasa (page 167) and repeat on the alternate leg.

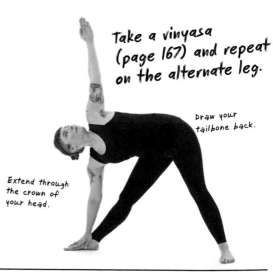

Draw your tailbone back.

Extend through the crown of your head.

4. REVERSE WARRIOR POSE (PAGE 86)

5. EXTENDED TRIANGLE POSE (PAGE 87)

STAND STRONG

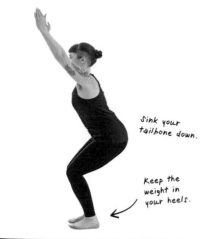

Sink your tailbone down.

Keep the weight in your heels.

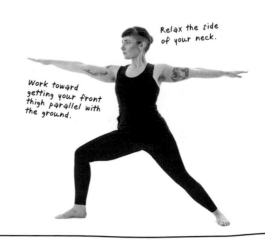

Relax the side of your neck.

Work toward getting your front thigh parallel with the ground.

2. CHAIR POSE (PAGE 82)

3. WARRIOR II (PAGE 84)

WHAT'S A VINYASA?

In a traditional vinyasa yoga practice, yoga sequences are separated by a transition called the *vinyasa*—it's actually a lot like a "mini Sun Salutation A." My favorite variation consists of:

High Plank (page 94) → Four-Limbed Staff Pose (page 96) or Half Chaturanga (page 96)

Half Chaturanga (page 96) → Cobra (page 116)

Cobra (page 116) or Upward-Facing Dog (page 117) → Downward-Facing Dog (page 80)

Feel free to insert this transition between your yoga sequences—as you pass from side to side and pose to pose, it will add a heightened fire to your body and take your practice to another level.

A CHICK-FIL-A BANDIT WALKS INTO WEIGHT WATCHERS

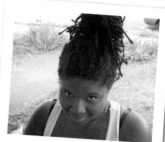

The face of a shameless french fry thief.

When I look back on it, I don't think I really gained an exorbitant amount of excess weight while I was in college. Sure, there were the requisite "freshman 15,"[18] but that was largely because the fast food I never attempted to avoid was now inescapable. UNC Greensboro's campus is cleverly outfitted with more than one fast-food kiosk, not to mention the off-campus haunts I frequented as often as possible. My college best friend and I would use my dining hall meal points to stock up on all the snack foods Tangela tried in vain to make me dislike as a kid. When my balance would run too low for the items we liked to buy, my friend and I would make a competitive game out of stealing Odwalla fruit smoothies and Chick-fil-A waffle fries as often as possible. Yes, that's right—in addition to being a lackadaisical college student, I had also become a bona fide Chick-fil-A waffle fry thief.

I really wish I could tell you that one day, after a particularly emotionally grating waffle fry burglary, I finally reached a point where ENOUGH WAS ENOUGH. In this alternate reality, College Jessamyn was tired of feeling lethargic and de-energized from all the stolen Chick-fil-A

---

18 Okay, let's just keep it real, it was much more like the freshman 50, but who's really counting?

fries. THIS version of College Jessamyn finally decided that she needed to change the way she thought about food.

Nah, bro. What can I say—College Jessamyn was a bitchy, self-entitled, whiny, Chick-fil-A-thieving suburbanite.

I could conceive of only one logical reason to change my ways and attempt a healthier lifestyle: I wanted to comfortably squeeze into Forever 21's size Large instead of having my fat rolls burst out of the fabric like a half-opened can of slice-and-bake biscuits. It was that simple.

> College Jessamyn was a bitchy, self-entitled, whiny, Chick-fil-A-thieving suburbanite.

With my best gal pals on board, I set out on a mission to "GET HEALTHY."[19] All of a sudden, I was retreating to the UNCG campus gym for late-night elliptical runs and spending my Saturday mornings slowly loping around the track while listening to Lady Gaga's *The Fame Monster* on repeat, dreaming of all the Forever 21 outfits I was finally going to be able to wear once I dropped at least a few dozen pounds from my staunchly size 18–20 body frame. I got my ass kicked at Zumba, became an occasional spin class attendee, and began to genuinely enjoy my time in the once-overwhelming weight room.[20]

But a halfhearted "obsession" with traditional exercise wasn't enough for my inner body-shaming Forever 21 Shopper. No, I needed to take it at least *one* step further. Along with three of my closest friends, I joined Weight Watchers during my junior year of college. I was intrigued by their unique method of tallying daily food goals—Weight Watchers uses a food "point" system as opposed to a traditional caloric counting system, so participants are somehow allowed to continue eating most of the same unhealthy food they'd been enjoying all along. For a lazy dieter like myself, it was basically a dream scenario.

---

19 What's an ill-fated health regimen without a fitness-related blood oath between close friends?

20 But let's be real, it was mostly because weight machines mean you can sit your ass down whenever you want.

For those of you who've never tried it, Weight Watchers is a lot like Alcoholics Anonymous, but you just substitute food for drinks and add a lot more scales and metaphors for compulsive eating. Here's how a typical Weight Watchers meeting circa 2008–2010 would go down:

At least once a week, you walk into the designated Weight Watchers reception/meeting room, which could be located in a somber office building or an equally somber church basement, depending on when you're able to make it to meetings. There's always lots of weight-loss-related paraphernalia available: food-tracking journals, point calculators, stacks of books about dealing with emotional eating. There's a reason Weight Watchers is a publicly traded company, and it's because those motherfuckers know how to hustle a weight-loss accessory.

Those motherfuckers know how to hustle a weight-loss accessory.

Once inside, you're shepherded into a line to have your weight recorded by one of the staff members. Weight Watchers staff positions were a coveted honor. In order to be hired as a receptionist or group leader, you have to actually *be* a Weight Watcher who has reached their goal weight. These Lifetime Weight Watchers always know exactly what to say when you step on or off the scale. For example, when you've lost weight, they basically start praise dancing in your honor and offering up encouraging, sisterly lines, like "YOU GO, CHICA! HALF A POUND LOST—YOU'RE GETTING SO CLOSE TO YOUR GOAL!"

However, when you've gained weight (my personal MO), they mask a disapproving frown behind a reassuring "Must have been a hard week, hon" or some other vaguely condescending sentiment. Elated by weight loss or blown to pieces by weight gain, you take a seat in a crowd of creaky folding chairs with your fellow Weight Watchers and nurse your ego. Once the whole group is assembled, animated group leaders drum up inspiring themed dialogue about the roadblocks between your current, unhealthy life and the future, healthy life you'll be free to live just as soon as you finally learn to resist nacho specials. This rousing discussion is always followed by an open forum portion, where members are encouraged to tell heart-wrenching tales from their weekly weight-loss struggle.

I actually loved that part of meetings. Food was one of my earliest addictions, and I found it extremely cathartic to sit in a room full of other food addicts and talk about the many ways I loved to disrespect my body. Before Weight Watchers, I'd never considered that there could be actual reasons for why I could never say no to an all-you-can-eat option. I had never really considered that there was a certain amount of personal responsibility, not to mention family history, at the root of my weird relationship with food.

For starters, my nuclear family was the utter definition of "working class." My parents married when they were absolute babies—my dad was twenty-one at their wedding and my mom, twenty-four, graduated from UNCG just a month prior to the big day. Tangela was pregnant by that fall, and I was born the following summer, just a few days after their first wedding anniversary. And when you get married straight out of college and happily—yet unexpectedly—acquire a baby barely one year later, no souls sprouting from that cabbage patch are floating to earth with silver spoons poking out of their mouths.

Even as an adult, I find purchasing expensive grocery items like individually wrapped string cheese and eight-ounce boxes of coconut water to be the absolute sign of financial prosperity. Because when I was a kid, Jesse and Tangela were not having any of that shit. My parents prided themselves in their financial frugality. They had to, frankly. My dad juggled two jobs, one at Sam's Club and another at UPS, in order to give his little clan the life he believed we deserved. And if my dad's job was to *make* the money, my mom's job was to spend that money carefully so we never had the lights turned off unexpectedly, ended up on food stamps, or got evicted. That meant managing every cent to the last inch of its life, which also meant that individually packaged

When you're raised in a family with limited means, it's a big deal to be in a situation where food is plentiful.

string cheese was some shit my brother and I only ate at a friend's house or on a field trip, but certainly not at our house on a regular-ass Thursday afternoon.

When you're raised in a family with limited means, it's a big deal to be in a situation where food is plentiful. On special occasions like family trips to visit my great-aunts in South Carolina or a birthday dinner at my favorite restaurant, Golden Corral, I was always encouraged by both my family and my inner Tiny Tim to eat as much as I absolutely could. I mean, let's be real—Stanley family holiday throwdowns weren't *entirely* like the Cratchit house on Christmas Day after Scrooge shows up, but it was certainly a luxury to have pans of macaroni and cheese at my disposal. It would have been deemed ridiculous by anyone in my family to only eat one serving of my favorite dishes when I could just as easily devour three. Same went for celebratory buffet dinners, except it was worse, because buffets add the additional requirement of *you better get your fucking money's worth.* I became accustomed to literally eating my heart out on every special occasion, be it Golden Corral birthday dinners, Bahá'í holy days, where heaps of traditional Persian food were standard fare, or academic award night pizza parties, which were never complete without me offering to polish off any extra slices my friends couldn't handle. Gluttony became a sign of decadent wealth, power, and happiness, even if it made me more overweight than I would have been otherwise.

Of course, I never discussed any of this during my Weight Watchers meetings. At Weight Watchers, I focused on the stereotypical suspects for weight gain: the fact that I was an overeating screwup who couldn't even manage to eat the amount of food that a regular 5-feet 6-inch woman should eat. "C'mon, Jessamyn," I'd silently berate myself. "Why can't you just eat three egg whites and a peach for breakfast without ending up in a fast-food drive-through before anyone's definition of a lunch hour? I mean, what the actual fuck is wrong with you?"

This mental flogging produced the expected results, and each of my (many) attempts at reaching my Weight Watchers goals always went down the exact same way: I would be a model Weight Watcher for the first few weeks—I'm talking pre-chopped carrot snack packs, Crock-Pots of lean ground chicken casseroles on deck, and a gym attendance record better than Tracy Anderson's. There might've even been kale smoothies going down, who knows? For me, the start of any health kick always felt as though I'd entered a state of holistic ecstasy. It was like drinking literal sunshine and shitting out metaphorical rainbows. Every inhale of oxygen was an opportunity to become the ~~healthy~~ THIN person buried inside myself.[21]

Of course, my resolve to live the healthiest life imaginable would always be thwarted by something. Maybe I would be particularly emotionally bolstered by a weekend of good sex with my college girlfriend—after all, if she loved my fat rolls, what difference did it make if we wolfed down two pizzas between two people? WHAT'S A PIZZA'S CALORIC COUNT IN THE FACE OF A PASSIONATE LESBIAN LOVE AFFAIR?

> The start of any health kick always felt as though I'd entered a state of holistic ecstasy.

Or maybe there would be a particularly outrageous party (or roster of parties) that needed to be attended? The social anxiety I'd harbored since childhood could be effectively neutralized with the right amount of alcohol, and god forbid I miss a chance to socialize with my peers in a beer-, wine-, and Everclear-drenched environment. Besides, my friends and I had a bunch of tricks we employed to lessen the effects of our alcohol-related caloric intake. What were our tricks, you ask? Well, like any college students worth their salt, our first step was to purposefully oversleep after a night of heavy drinking. This is a critical step, as it allows your functional alcoholic Weight Watcher to sleep away most of the typical "eating hours" in a given day. When I'd drag myself out of bed, I'd try to

---

21 Because, let's be real, the Western definition of the word healthy has somehow become completely synonymous with the Western definition of the word thin.

eat a "healthy" option—maybe an unreasonably large salad coated in ranch dressing and bacon fat.

Then perhaps I'd shuffle off to the gym in order to lazily jog off a maximum of two of the prior evening's innumerable beers. By that time it would be logical to start getting ready for another night of partying, and I'd try to drink as much water as possible during this pre-party prep time in order to "get in my daily water count," aka "lubricate my liver for all the liquor to come." My friends and I would then proceed to have a repeat performance of the previous evening—drinking at various locations and with an ever-changing cast of guest stars until the wee hours, walking each other home, and praying that the Weight Watchers scale would somehow fail to calculate the slew of inevitable empty calories being ingested.

In any case, I can't deny that my inability to refuse a cheap/free/ available drink was a huge contributor to my Weight Watchers failures.

After attending a few weigh-ins and getting the curt death stare of doom from my resident receptionists and group leaders because of my obvious unraveling of commitment, I would become too embarrassed by my perceived failures to continue attending meetings. Instead of recommitting to Weight Watchers with increased fervor and sticking out my considerable weight-loss plateaus, I would suddenly become way too busy to attend regular meetings and allow my weight to freely spike once again.

I wonder what would have happened if I'd asked all the right questions of myself at Weight Watchers.

Only once did I reach an actual weight loss peak. Right before my undergraduate graduation, I managed to lose nearly thirty pounds. Finally, after years of effort, I was able to comfortably wear a solid size 16 and (sort of) fit into a Forever 21 size Large. Because of my hard-won success, I figured I could handle the difficulty of independent weight loss without continuing to give Weight Watchers a stiff monthly membership fee. I finished college and entered graduate school with a new lease on life, a daily biking schedule, and a commitment to eating all the foods that *Self* magazine tells us to eat. However, my resolve wasn't nearly as strong as I had thought, and it wasn't long before I slipped back into my old patterns and gained back all of the weight I'd lost.

Sometimes I wonder what would have happened if I'd asked all the right questions of myself at Weight Watchers. What if I'd asked myself WHY I felt compelled to overeat, WHY I couldn't stop binge drinking, and WHY I constantly fought a hatred for physical exercise? I probably could've mended wounds that have festered since childhood and actually stuck to a lifelong dietary and exercise change.

But then again, I probably would've pulled a Jennifer Hudson, lost a million pounds, never started practicing yoga, and never had a reason to write this book, and my life would more than likely be completely different. Sooooo ultimately I'm kinda glad that Weight Watchers and I were never a true match made in heaven.

LESSON LEARNED

I could never seem to find balance back in those Chick-fil-A thievin', Weight Watchin' days. I was either eating too much, obsessing about weight loss too much, drinking (*WAY*) too much, or involved in some other equally unfortunate and unhealthy mix of activities. And honestly, when I see my students struggle with poses like Extended Hand to Big Toe (page 92), I wonder if they have struggles with balance in their own lives. That's usually how things work—if you can't find balance in your life, balance on the mat is hard to come by. Start practicing the following sequence if you struggle with balance in your life—usually, if we can capture a sense of balance on the mat, it will resonate to the other parts of our lives that need a little help.

I NEED TO FEE

Begin with three rounds of
Sun Salutation A (page 144) and
either: I Want to Stand Strong
(page 166) or one to two rounds
of Sun Salutation B (page 148)

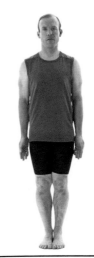

1. MOUNTAIN POSE (PAGE 74)

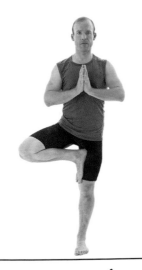

4. TREE POSE (PAGE 89)

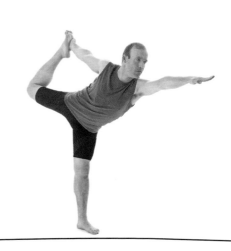

5. DANCER POSE (PAGE 90)

BALANCED

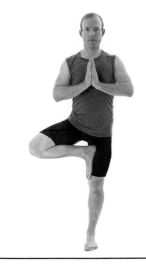

2. TREE POSE (PAGE 89)

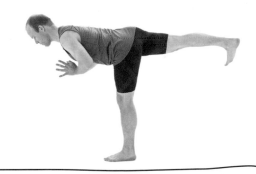

3. WARRIOR III (PAGE 85)

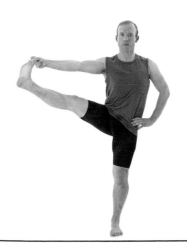

**6. EXTENDED HAND TO BIG TOE
(PAGE 92)**

Take a vinyasa (page 167) and
repeat on the alternate leg.

TABOR CITY FUNERALS

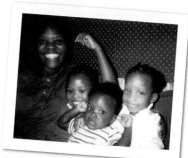

Aunt Tiriah, cousins Brooke, Myles, and your truly, circa 1990

By summer 2012, I'd been practicing Bikram yoga for a hot minute—over time, it became my salvation. It restored me in ways that I never knew to desire, and I was just starting to consistently feel good about myself again. And, after enduring a pretty intense breakup with my high school sweetheart the previous year, I had a new girlfriend in my orbit, and I was ready to make even bigger changes in my life. My new girlfriend had recently relocated to Durham and, because I'm nothing if not a walking lesbian cliché, I dropped out of graduate school and followed her to Durham in the summer of 2012.

Oh, don't give me that look—I'm sure you've done worse things for love. Yeah, I'm talking to you, person who was married and divorced by their thirtieth birthday. Oh, and by the way, leisurely and flippantly dropping into conversation that I "dropped out of graduate school" couldn't be a more understated way of describing an atomic-level bombshell in my life.[22] However, I knew that the changes I needed were not going to happen in Winston-Salem. I felt that I'd made a foolhardy decision by deciding

---

22 I'm not an academic quitter, and it's for a good reason—my father dropped out of college to get married and always regretted the decision. I will never forget the chill in his voice when I told him of my decision to leave my program. He said not finishing grad school would be the mistake of my life. He may have been as pissed at me as he still was at himself.

to rush into my graduate education, and the move to Durham felt like an opportunity to re-navigate my life. And so, with fear and trepidation, I took a temporary withdrawal from graduate school, packed up my shit, and started bouncing between my parents' couch and my girlfriend's tiny apartment while she and I looked for a space big enough for two. Of course, this was no small feat—in addition to the fact that I was painfully broke, I still needed to find a job. And as anyone who has ever been without a job will tell you, looking for a job is a full-time job of its own. I was reeling from all of the changes in my life, but desperate to keep my chin up.

Certain things stick out to me about the day my aunt died. It was the middle of July and, like most summer days in the state of North Carolina, it was stiflingly hot. That day, my girlfriend and I had arranged to view an apartment in my favorite historic apartment building in Durham. It's a beautiful building that still stops me in my tracks. And it was exclusive as all hell—the kind of spot where you had to "know someone" in order to secure a viewing. The whole process of "getting in" to the building had been dicey, uncertain, and time-consuming, so my girlfriend and I were thrilled when the manager got back in touch to say that there was in fact a two-bedroom unit available in our price range, and could we come see it as soon as possible? We hauled ass over to the building, parked in the tiny private lot—and that's when my phone rang. I was in such a great mood that I almost didn't believe my mother when she said that my aunt Tiriah had passed away an hour or so before.

It didn't seem possible. I mean, not to be hyperbolic, but my aunt Tiriah was a motherfucking monster.[23] You know how there are people that you think will never die? For me, several people have rested on this list (Michael Jackson, Prince, Amy Winehouse), and, in the blood relative category, my aunt Tiriah was definitely one of the headliners. Tiriah Scott was one of the liveliest and most robust women I've ever known, and she

---

23 No, this isn't the same aunt I mentioned earlier—this isn't the aunt who took me to my first yoga class. Damn, this story would be even more tragic if it were the same aunt, wouldn't it? They're both my mother's sisters. And their names are Tiriah and Tracy. Yes, all their names start with a T. Is that enough synergy for you?

seemed completely invincible. She was a woman of endless talents and abilities. A Martha Stewart–level domestic goddess, an elementary school teacher, a proud military wife and mother. She was in every organization, belonged to every club. She was ridiculously smart and one of the most driven people I've ever known—even though she became pregnant with my eldest cousin when she was fresh out of high school and had two more children shortly thereafter, she never stopped trying to finish her college education. She'd finished college after her fortieth birthday, long after we'd all stopped believing she'd graduate. She leaped all of these hurdles with a rueful grin—she was known for her infectious sense of humor and vivaciousness. She was my role model in every way, a pillar of strength, and absolutely invincible.

She was my role model in every way, a pillar of strength, and absolutely invincible.

No, my mom must have been confused. Aunt Tiriah couldn't possibly be gone.

But she was. At the age of forty-five, Tiriah had collapsed while doing a load of laundry. My grandma Marvella was the one who discovered her body.

I was no stranger to death. I'd donned black garb for hordes of distant family members, but I'd never experienced death and loss on such an intimate level. I grew up in a very insulated and tight-knit family that exhibited the model of "it takes a village to raise a child." My mother's relationships with her sisters and my grandmother were a thickly woven part of our family's tapestry and overall survival. While probably not quite in line with Norman Rockwell's depiction of the "all-American family," this kind of matriarchy is common in black American families. I think it's the result of the fact that so many black American families were ripped apart by the effects of slavery, and matriarchal communal family rearing was a naturally occurring survival technique.

My auntie and I were tight from the moment I came out of the womb. When I was born, Tiriah picked me up out of my mother's arms and proclaimed that I absolutely must be *her* child because I looked just like her. My mom thought she had a point—after all, I'd come out of the womb sporting a chubby neck dressed with juicy fat rolls, a distinctive physical feature that only my aunt Tiriah possessed. I still remember taking baths and showers with my aunt when I was a little girl—she was the person who taught me how to properly "clean my clam," as she always called it. Even when she wasn't physically near, she always felt close by.

Many of my actions and natural abilities mimicked hers, and I'd been trying to nail down her comic timing since childhood. She really was hilarious—she could make anyone laugh, at the drop of a hat, simply by being herself. She and I even had the exact same weird toe size distribution—both of our first toes are oddly longer than any of our other toes. She was, in short, an irreplaceably large part of my genesis. Her passing was a reminder of mortality in a very brutal way. It wasn't as though she'd suffered a long illness or lived a life of crime wherein unexpected death wasn't all that unexpected. She was just living her regular life. She was doing a load of laundry, for Chrissake.

I'm not much for tearful displays of emotion. Even when I was being bullied in grade school, I never cried in front of my enemies. I learned to hide my feelings then, and I carried that ability like a shield of armor. This moment was no exception. I rushed off the phone with my mom, consoling her as much as I could without alarming my girlfriend who, of course, was sitting patiently next to me, waiting to view an apartment that I suddenly couldn't care less about at all. But as soon as I got off the phone, I steeled myself. Internally, I was completely devastated. But somehow, thanks to years of holding in my tears and hiding my emotions, I hadn't begun to externally process my pain—thereby making it much easier to simply *distract* myself from the pain. I was left with two options: I could bail on the apartment viewing and rush to my parents' house in Jamestown to start our version of a black American shivah, or I could pretend as though nothing had happened and go view my (maybe) dream apartment.

It was then that I reminded myself of my aunt Tiriah's trademark pragmatism—specifically as it pertained to the ancient art of bargain shopping and getting the absolute best deal available. This was a woman who would never let a dope apartment pass her by, grieving period or no grieving period. This was a lady who knew the value of an affordable rent in the right zip code.

This was a lady who knew the value of an affordable rent in the right zip code.

I imagined my auntie settling herself into the backseat of my girlfriends's car, legal pad in hand, ready to help me ponder the right decision. So I made the decision she would have made—I pretended everything was fine and went to view the apartment. And I have to confess, I really think she would have been *extremely* proud of that decision. I mean, in what alternate reality would the flesh and blood of Tiriah Scott pass up an amazing, F. Scott Fitzgeraldian Art Deco apartment, simply to cry and grieve? Bitch, please.

I returned home for the funeral. By the time my aunt passed away, I'd attended more funerals than weddings, baptisms, and religious revivals combined. And that's saying a lot, considering I grew up in a devout religious family smack dab in the middle of the Bible Belt—baptisms, weddings, and revivals are big business in our neck of the woods. But bad nutrition and undiagnosed chronic health problems are also big business, and so funerals are a frequent style of family gathering. My family was all too comfortable with planning and gathering for funerals in Tabor City, the minuscule East Carolinian hamlet that doubles as our family mother ship. But this was one Tabor City funeral that left an unforgettable impression on yours truly.

My entire family was falling apart in the wake of her death, and there wasn't very much space for me to feel anything during the service. My mother is a big emoter—it's possible that Tangela was a chest-beating, hair-pulling, Greco-Roman widow in a past life. My grandmother was completely overcome by grief, and I'm fairly certain that the memory of finding her once-healthy but now very much dead child on the floor of a suburban basement never left Marvella's line of sight . . . well, maybe ever.[24]

But loud grief has never been my style, and I've always used jokes as a way to ease tension. In this case, however, laughter just covered up my sadness. Each joke just masked my endless darkness. I couldn't believe she'd left us. I couldn't believe I'd been so emotionally unprepared. I couldn't believe how much I was hurting. And I didn't know who to talk to about it. My parents were so wrapped up in their own grief that I couldn't possibly try to share it with them. My brother and my cousins were all so far away in their own respective solar systems, and it seemed bizarre to try to bring our solar systems into orbit. And while I loved my girlfriend very much, ours was not a relationship built on open-ended conversations about death and the nature of life. I felt

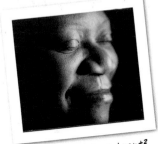

wasn't my granny a beaut?

very much adrift, and when I returned home to Durham and started trying to rebuild my life in the combined wreckage of both my mid-twenties crisis and my aunt's passing, I found my explanation for life's meaning to be wanting.

Not to mention the fact that, at the time of my aunt's death, my yoga practice wasn't in the best shape. My absence of income and need to secure indoor housing meant I had no spare cash for yoga classes. When I was living in Winston-Salem and still somehow managing to drag my thoroughly uninspired ass into my grad school classes, I took advantage of the Winston-Salem Bikram studio's really dope payment option: You could practice for free as long as you attended classes four to five times every week

---

24 My grandmother was deeply traumatized by my aunt's passing. She'd been diagnosed with diabetes a number of years before, but she completely let her health go by the wayside after Aunt Tiriah died. Her health gradually declined over the next year, and in fall 2013, she also passed away. Like my aunt, she played a massive role in my upbringing. She lived with my nuclear family for large chunks of my childhood and adolescence, and my grief over her passing is still relatively fresh and, therefore, occasionally very overwhelming.

and helped clean the studios after class. It was the perfect option, and it meant that I was able to practice all the time—much more than I would've been able to practice otherwise.

But I soon learned that the work-study program at my beloved Winston-Salem studio was the mystical unicorn of yoga payment options.

I was losing both my yoga practice and my emotional clarity.

My new local Bikram studio in Durham had no work-study program and was twice as expensive. Since I'd decided to put myself in a financial tailspin by leaving the magical land of student loan refund checks, I was in nowhere near the financial position to start paying nearly $15 every time I wanted to take a yoga class.[25]

I was crestfallen, but I tried to convince myself that going to class every once in a while would be exactly the same as going to class nearly every day. It's not. And with every missed class, my body began to lose a little of the elasticity it had gained over the previous year of regular practice. I began to feel myself slipping—I was losing both my yoga practice and my emotional clarity. Frankly, I was just having a really fucking rough summer. My aunt's passing, my decision to leave grad school—it was all becoming too much to handle. I knew I needed to do something or else the next solution would be a psychiatrist's office and (inevitably) a prescription for antidepressants and antianxiety meds.

LESSON LEARNED

I doubt my home yoga practice would exist if my aunt hadn't died. Prior to her passing, I had never practiced without the watchful gaze of a Bikram teacher. For one thing, I thought I couldn't practice without a teacher telling me whether I was endangering myself with bad alignment. And while I'd

---

25 Here's a tip for all twentysomethings—don't drop out of grad school when you don't have any savings and still have to repay student loans for a degree you don't actively intend to complete.

always been capable of harvesting a fair amount of athletic masochism, I'd never had a motivator outside of pure physical enjoyment to keep me on the path of athletic activity.[26]

My aunt's death literally turned my life upside down. But, in spite of the fact that my grief has never really subsided, her passing helped me accept that it's sometimes very necessary to see the world from another angle. Inversions offer us a way to strengthen our bodies in a number of different ways—among other things, they work our core strength, shoulder conditioning, and hamstring flexibility. Above all else, inversions provide us with an opportunity to quite literally turn our worlds upside down and see things from a completely different perspective. Progress on this sequence might come slowly—that's okay. Take your time, don't rush, and practice this sequence over and over again. True strength doesn't magically appear overnight—it comes as the result of hard work, sweat, and (more than likely) tears. Embrace the process, accept the gift of slow progress, and revel in an opportunity to truly see the world from another angle.

---

26 Athletic nuts often fall on the spectrum of masochists. Self-flagellation wears many coats, y'all.

I WANT TO SEE
FROM

Begin with either I Want to Stand Strong (page 166) or I Need to Feel Balanced (page 176)

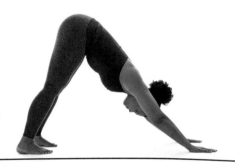

1. DOWNWARD-FACING DOG (PAGE 80)

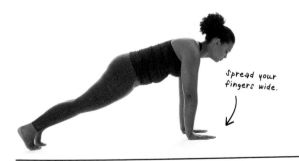

Spread your fingers wide.

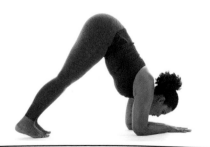

4. HIGH PLANK (PAGE 94)

5. DOLPHIN POSE (PAGE 99)

THE WORLD ANOTHER ANGLE

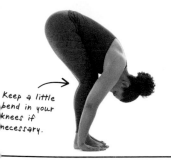

Keep a little bend in your knees if necessary.

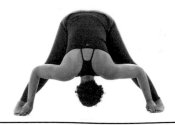

2. STANDING FORWARD FOLD (PAGE 76)

3. WIDE-LEGGED FORWARD BEND (PAGE 97)

Flex through the soles of your feet.

Draw your thighs together.

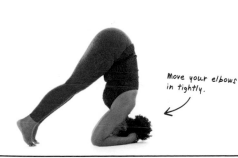

Move your elbows in tightly.

Take a vinyasa (page 167) and repeat steps 1—7.

6. SUPPORTED HEADSTAND PREP (PAGE 101)

7. SUPPORTED HEADSTAND (PAGE 101)

A YOGA PRACTICE GROWS IN DURHAM

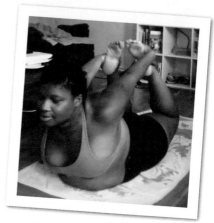

One of my first yoga selfies

I was scared as hell to practice yoga at home. I'd literally never practiced outside of a studio before. I mean, there was no one there to tell me if what I was doing was right . . . wasn't that required? Bikram classes had led me to believe an instructor's presence was absolutely necessary in order to practice. But I told myself that as long as I was practicing poses with which I already had a passing familiarity, I could practice safely in my living room.[27]

I couldn't have anticipated that I would fall madly in love with the simple pleasure of practicing yoga at home. I mean, it would be impossible for me to tell you how happy I felt when I started practicing yoga all by my lonesome. It was one of the most freeing things I've ever done in my life. Everything about the way I was practicing yoga felt unorthodox, and it was exciting. For the first time, I was free to wear whatever I wanted, hold poses as long as I wanted, and break a lot of rules.

Up until that point, I'd never tried to practice yoga without staring

---

27 I will never understand why everyone walks into yoga class with a chronic fear of practicing the poses incorrectly. It's like one wrong step will kill you. I mean, we will ride in airplanes, or eat food that's essentially rat poison, and no one bats an eye. But suggest that a novice yoga practitioner tackle a foundational asana on their own without an alignment-focused instructor's eye and it's like you've suggested self-mutilation.

at the other people in the room. I'd always used my fellow students as the barometer for what I should be doing, but without other people present, I felt infinitely more comfortable. I felt free to fall down, because there was no one there to see me when I hit the ground. So I started allowing myself to fall without judgment. That process allowed me the freedom to try out poses from the Bikram sequence that I'd been too self-conscious to *really* try out in a class full of people. All of a sudden, poses like Dancer Pose (page 90), which had been almost completely out of my reach in the past, were finally feeling accessible.

There were still times when I wasn't quite sure if I was practicing the poses correctly. I'd fret over my foot placement or hip alignment, and I wasn't sure what to do about it. Like any self-respecting millennial, I took to the internet to find answers to my alignment questions. I remember being mesmerized by the resources available to me after 0.125 seconds on Google. My knowledge of asana was very limited by Bikram's meager 26 postures, and I found myself falling like Alice into a yogic wonderland.

While I enjoyed the polished, professional video yoga tutorials, I quickly found that the best yoga resources were in amateur-level still photography on a fledgling app called Instagram. At the time, Instagram was still a pretty niche social media app. I'd been using it for about a year, but it hadn't been around much longer than that, and it seemed to only really have traction with millennials in my age range. I was surprised to find a community of yoga people on Instagram, and I was seriously impressed by all the poses they could pull off that I'd never seen before. The most helpful pictures were selfies from regular hobbyist yoga practitioners like myself who were looking for feedback on their progress. There were even Instagram yoga challenges where people practiced a series of poses over the course of the month and posted a photo every day.

I was free to wear whatever I wanted, hold poses as long as I wanted, and break a lot of rules.

Initially, I just stared at the poses in wonder. I wasn't in any rush to photograph my own progress. I didn't feel confident enough in my ability to think my poses were worthy of being photographed, and my apprehension over practicing yoga in front of mirrors definitely extended to cameras as well. Eventually, I began researching the preparatory postures recommended for some of the more advanced poses I wanted to try. I spent a considerable amount of time perusing *Yoga Journal*'s print and online editions, learning about new poses, and when the time was right, I just started gradually working some of those preparatory postures into my little homegrown Bikram-esque sequence.

Over time, my understanding of flow yoga grew to the point where I felt comfortable challenging myself well out of comfort zones I'd predetermined long ago. I found myself practicing poses that became progressively more difficult than anything I'd tried in the past. I finally became confident enough to post my own pictures. This all happened at home, alone, in a little corner of a 750-square-foot apartment that I shared with my ex-girlfriend, a rambunctious pit-mix, and my grouchy orange tabby cat. It was a type of self-examination I'd never undertaken and that completely changed the way I viewed myself. I was finally on my way to the goal drilled into every Bikram student—becoming my own true teacher.

LESSON LEARNED

Without my home yoga practice, I would never have started photographing my asana practice. I probably wouldn't have ever started teaching yoga. My home practice really did energize my spirit, and offered me a profoundly different outlook on life that wouldn't have been possible otherwise.

A simple infusion of new energy and activity in your life can make an incredible impact on the condition of your spirit. The yogic equivalent of an energy booster is a backbend—they rip open your central nervous system and send energy coursing through your body. It's natural to feel like you've "seen stars" when you're practicing backbends. Take time to absorb each backbend pose after you've practiced it—absorption and contemplation are just as important (if not more important) than physical action.

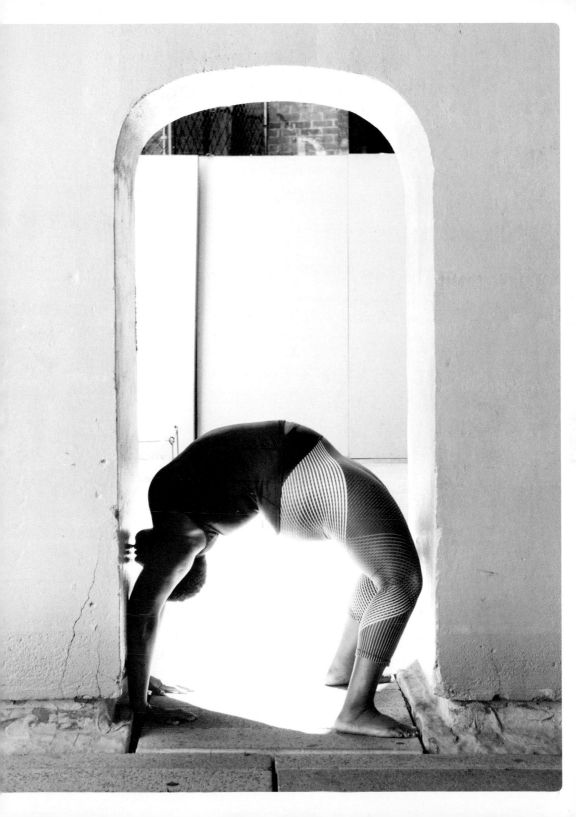

I WANT TO ENEF

Begin with either I Want to Stand Strong (page 166), I Need to Feel Balanced (page 176), I Want to See the World from Another Angle (page 186), or I Need to Release Fear (page 200)

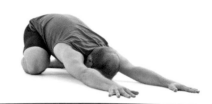

I. CHILD'S POSE (PAGE 124)

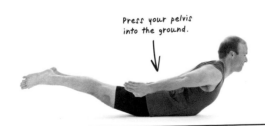

Press your pelvis into the ground.

4. LOCUST (PAGE 118)

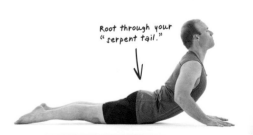

Root through your "serpent tail."

5. COBRA (PAGE 116)

SIZE MY SPIRIT

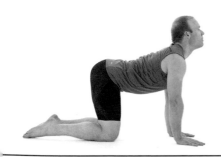

2. CAT/COW POSE (PAGE 114)

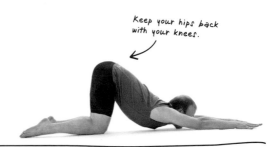

Keep your hips back with your knees.

3. EXTENDED PUPPY DOG POSE (PAGE 115)

Take a vinyasa (page 167) and repeat sequence.

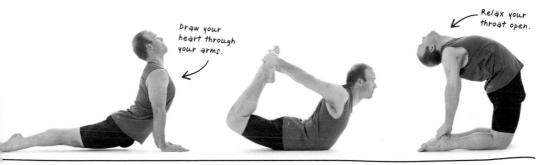

Draw your heart through your arms.

Relax your throat open.

6. UPWARD-FACING DOG (PAGE 117)

7. BOW POSE (PAGE 119)

8. CAMEL POSE (PAGE 120)

SELF-ACCEPTANCE: THE TABOO

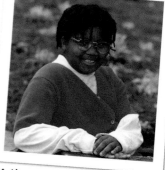

Self-acceptance was hard to come by in my Harry Potter glasses days.

Accepting our bodies is the most crucial aspect of holistic health and happiness—and a strong yoga practice. But it can be really effing hard to reconcile the realities of our anatomy with the delusions of our mind. I've always wanted to be dainty, but I'm genetically burly. My shoulders are broad as all hell—I am truly my father's daughter. In yoga, it's really important to understand your body's actual foundation—shoulders, hips, wrists, and elbows all must be in proper alignment. And if you place your hands and arms too close together because you don't wish to accept your shoulders' actual width, you will have jacked-up alignment every time. When I began practicing yoga, I completely misunderstood my shoulder girdle size and found it extremely difficult to hold basic yoga poses like Downward-Facing Dog, High Plank, and Four-Limbed Staff Pose. Basically, it was damn near impossible for me to find a stable foundation in yoga asana because of my inability to accept my body's natural structure. However, once I found a way to accept my body's structure, my whole perspective of asana practice shifted for the better.

When I see companies attempting to package and distribute "body positivity," I always have to fight off rounds of the giggles. I mean, they try to package self-acceptance as something you can purchase at your local shopping center, right next to face masks and laxatives. I think we can all agree that shit doesn't really work that way. First of all, can we acknowledge for a moment that corporate America is basically the source of body negativity? Think about how much companies profit when you feel shitty about yourself. I mean, if we thought our skin was perfect exactly as it is, would we feel compelled to buy Dove's latest face cream? If we thought our lips were perfect as they are, would we look twice at Maybelline's new lip color line?

No, we wouldn't.

I can only speak for myself, but my early life's ambition was to embody whatever beauty ideals were being perpetuated by the most popular and loudest voices. And if you don't fit within their *very* narrow definition of beauty, you're expected to change every detail of yourself until you *do* fit in the definition.

> *It can be really effing hard to reconcile the realities of our anatomy with the delusions of our mind.*

And yeah, this isn't just an issue for people who call themselves women—men have just as much body dysmorphia as ladies. In some cases, it's definitely way worse.[28] And when we only let one category of people call all the mental shots, the only way for things to go is badly.

I'll be damned if there's a public space we can enter without throwing painful barbs at ourselves and others—whether it's a middle-aged mom who refuses a slice of chocolate cake because she's "already too fat," a teenage girl who deems a fellow Forever 21 shopper "too chunky for that top," or a barrel-chested guy who hesitates to participate in a 5K because "other people shouldn't have to see man boobs jiggling around." All of these words create a toxic language that pollutes the way we see ourselves and those around us.

I've never observed a scene where toxic body language is as widespread and generally accepted as within the fitness world. In pursuit of health

---

28 / mean, I have major sympathy for guys—imagine if the only kind of athletic body you were allowed to idolize was a cross between Channing Tatum and Ryan Reynolds. At least femmebots have the thick thighs of Serena Williams to openly idolize with abandon. Damn. It's hard in the streets for the boys.

and well-being, most athletic arenas become festering breeding grounds for negative body language. You would think that the Modern yoga world would be a relatively safe space, free of sizephobia and judgment, but that is far from reality.

Let's take a look at "Jill," a thirty-six-year-old mother of two, her body curvier and more "structurally unique" than she remembers it pre-pregnancy. (In my yoga classes, I meet quite a few Jills. Maybe you're a Jill too.) As Jill stares at her fellow yoga practitioners rolling out their mats before class, she admires their sinewy arms and laser-cut abdomens and immediately begins berating herself for not resembling them. She thinks, "I need to lose at least twenty pounds. How am I going to make it through this yoga class if I don't look like them?"

By giving voice to this hateful body language, Jill is creating two problems:

First of all, she's ruining her opportunity for a pleasurable yoga practice. By deciding that her body is somehow unsuitable for yoga, our heroine has poisoned her brain, the one muscle that can truly make or break her potential for a soothing practice. It's likely that this perfectly capable and strong woman (she gave birth to two children, for crying out loud) will underestimate her abilities and allow the phrase "I can't" to define her practice.

Second of all, let's say our heroine decides to share some of her body hate spiel with one of her fellow classmates. Not only has she poisoned *her* brain with judgment, but she's also poisoned the mind and mood of her friend. Instead of adding to the positive vibe of her yoga studio, she's now become an active participant in an unspoken hierarchy where certain bodies matter and others don't. Without recognizing it, Jill has inadvertently assumed the role of her own oppressor.

At what point would YOU finally say, "I've had enough of hating my body"?

At what point would YOU finally say, "I've had enough of hating my body"? Accepting our bodies is more than just size acceptance. It's understanding that beneath these layers of complicated fabric, we're all basically the same. Imperfect (yet absolutely perfect) humans.

I didn't understand my body unhappiness for the majority of my life, and I believed what the media told me—I assumed my body was built incorrectly and desperately hoped to wake up one day looking like someone else. Instead of seeking out the core of my dislike, I chose to hide myself behind my clothes, makeup, and hair extensions. I happily took any route I could find to resemble the picture of beauty presented to me in movies, magazines, and TV shows. I know I'm not the only person who has felt this way—we want to be accepted by our peers, and the pursuit of peer acceptance results in a desperate (and ultimately futile) struggle to don someone else's skin.

If our lives truly revolve around *acceptance*, why don't we focus that same amount of energy on *SELF-acceptance*? So many doctors immediately disregard self-acceptance in favor of facts and figures about scientifically accepted healthy body composition. Sometimes it feels like the entire Western medical profession believes losing weight and maintaining a body size that's defined as "healthy" is the single route to happiness. I hope I'm not the only person who finds this argument laughable. We all struggle with debilitating emotional boundaries. Bad self-esteem and body shame know no size—they happen to everyone. What makes the difference is how we choose to handle our self-esteem issues and body shame—do we accept them or allow free rein over all our judgments?

Honestly, body discrimination doesn't end even when you become a yoga teacher. I can't tell you the number of people who have walked into my yoga classes completely shocked and confused to see me sitting behind the check-in counter. They usually smile curtly and ask if I'm the teacher or merely checking people in. When I cheerfully reply that yes, I'm actually the teacher, I can clearly see their faces flash from "WHAT THE ACTUAL FUCK" to "Dammit, I guess I'm gonna have to pay this fat girl $15 to get a lackluster exercise experience." It should be no surprise that most people think fat people have no idea how to lead an exercise class.[29] It takes

---

29 Ironically, those are usually the same students who have sweat dripping from their eyeballs and are winded about halfway through the class.

confidence to accept ourselves exactly as we are in the face of people who want us to doubt our abilities. It means realizing that we're really dealing with fear—we're afraid of being judged.

LESSON LEARNED

Fear can take a physical toll. If our bodies are outfitted with a stress storage bin, our hips fit the bill. Every time we feel compelled to flee or fight in our daily lives, our reactions become trapped in our hip joints. By releasing and relaxing our hips on a regular basis, especially with sequences like the one that follows, we can unburden ourselves of the emotional weights that make it difficult to move forward and be present in life. If you find that this sequence brings up unexpected emotions, just embrace them. By unburdening your hips of tension you can unburden the space around your heart and allow yourself to be more present, calm, and happy on a daily basis.

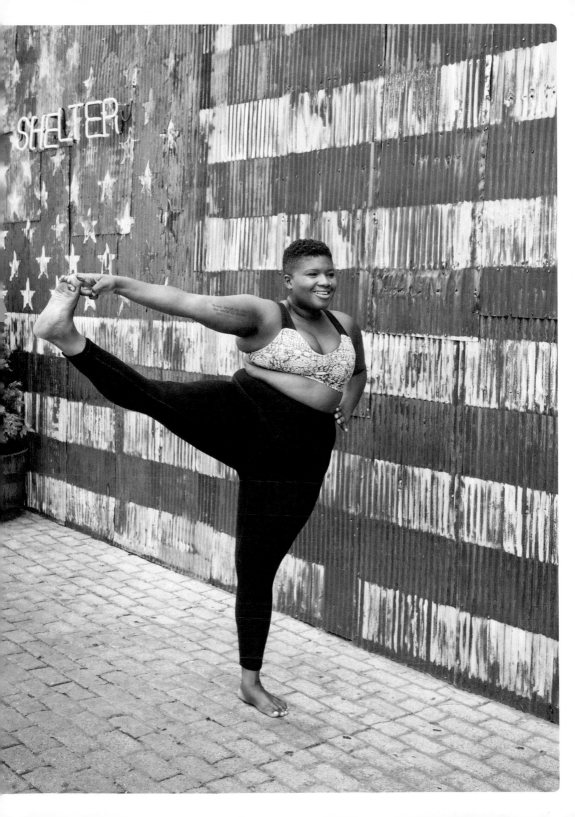

I NEED TO

Begin with either I Want to Stand Strong (page 166), I Need to Feel Balanced (page 176), or I Want to See the World from Another Angle (page 186).

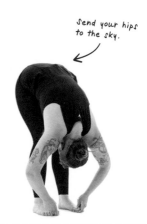

Send your hips to the sky.

I. BIG TOE HOLD (PAGE 77)

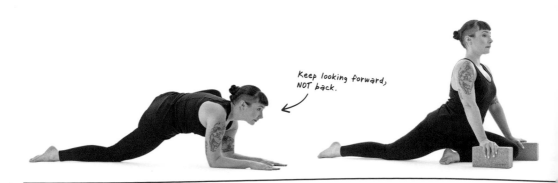

Keep looking forward, NOT back.

5. LIZARD LUNGE POSE (PAGE 107)

6. ONE-LEGGED KING PIGEON POSE (SUPPORTED, PAGE 110)

RELEASE FEAR

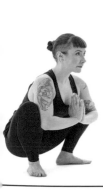

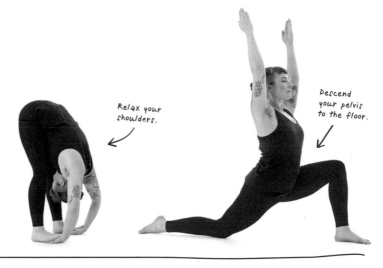

Relax your shoulders.

Descend your pelvis to the floor.

2. GARLAND POSE (PAGE 104)

3. HAND UNDER FOOT (PAGE 77)

4. HIGH/LOW LUNGE (PAGES 105 AND 106)

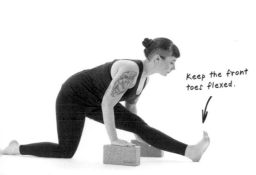

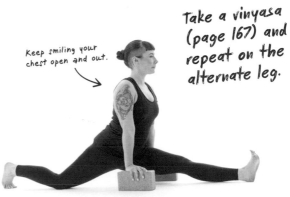

Keep the front toes flexed.

Keep smiling your chest open and out.

Take a vinyasa (page 167) and repeat on the alternate leg.

7. RUNNER'S LUNGE (SUPPORTED, PAGE 108)

8. MONKEY POSE (SUPPORTED, PAGE 113)

THE SCARLET A

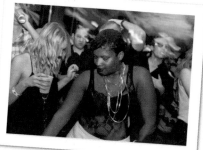

TRUE LIFE: I used to be a party girl.

Once, on a very chilly, very early Sunday morning, a Durham County police officer found me asleep at the wheel of my beat-up Honda Accord. It was a few months before my twenty-seventh birthday, and I'd fallen asleep on my way home from work. It was two a.m.—what was typically a very congested intersection was bare as a bone, and my car was still chugging away. Mr. Nice Cop kindly nudged me awake and asked if I would exit the vehicle. Once I did as he asked, Mr. Nice Cop politely asked if he could administer a field sobriety test.

Of course, polite Southern femme that I am, I agreed. I passed the balance tests with flying colors—my regular work on yoga poses like Extended Hand to Big Toe (page 92) meant standing on one leg and heel-toeing a line was a breeze, and my only real qualm with the whole procedure was that my outfit wasn't particularly conducive to impromptu outdoor activities. I was wearing a very short red miniskirt and a sleeveless, partially backless white top—while it'd been a perfectly appropriate outfit for hauling ass through a steaming-hot restaurant for hours on end, it wasn't really ideal attire for North Carolina's frigid early spring mornings.

Unfortunately, balance tests are not the only component of a field sobriety test. As soon as the officer pulled out the infamous Breathalyzer machine and (still, politely) asked if I would please blow into the straw, my blood started to race a little harder than before.

You see, I *was* drunk. That's precisely why I'd fallen asleep at the wheel of my car in an empty intersection at two o'clock in the morning. Yeah, sure, I'd fed Mr. Nice Cop a mumbled explanation that I'd fallen asleep because I was exhausted from work, which was absolutely true. My work schedule consisted of day and night shifts at two different jobs, and my exhaustion was palpable. But I'd actually *fallen asleep* because, yeah—I was drunk. I'd spent the two hours prior to last call downing a combination of wine, beer, and Fireball shots with my coworkers and friends, after which I'd made the conscious decision to drive home.

Drinking became the key to unlocking my emotional vault.

Of course, I didn't have to tell Mr. Nice Cop any of those details—the Breathalyzer test did that part for me. I wasn't really all that surprised when he charged me with a DWI/DUI and I ended up spending a night in jail—after all, I'd been aware of my alcohol problem for years.

My parents had done everything they could to prevent this from happening. The Bahá'í faith encourages complete abstinence from drugs and alcohol; my parents were and continue to be staunch teetotalers.[30] If drinking or related activities came up in conversation, my parents always took care and time to discourage my brother and me from ever imbibing. Alcohol abstinence and avoidance was the Stanley family rule, with absolutely no exception.

I started drinking for all the same cliché reasons teenagers and twentysomethings have consumed alcohol since the beginning of time: It was forbidden and it felt good. As I grew older, liquor, wine, and beer became the magical cure for my social anxiety, and I was amazed by how quickly a few drinks could provide relief from stress. And because I'd never received any alcohol education beyond my parents' "just say no" approach, I

---

30 That and the fact that my maternal grandfather was a storied abusive alcoholic. His relationship with my mother was so terrible that he was absent for most of my early life—in the end, I only met him once before he passed away.

had no idea what it meant to drink responsibly. Things definitely worsened after the deaths of my aunt Tiriah and my grandmother—I was unable to fully process my emotions, and drinking became the key to unlocking my emotional vault.

By the time I ended up in a Durham County holding cell, I'd logged years of extreme drinking, and I wasn't at all surprised to see where my choices had led. As I sat on the concrete floor, nursing a throbbing headache and a mouth that felt like it'd been washed out with cotton wool, I started asking myself a series of unpleasant questions. Did the fact that I'd been arrested mean I was an alcoholic? Did I need to start going to AA? Was I going to get out of jail in time to work my next shift at the restaurant? And, most important, what the fuck was wrong with me?

It took me a while to figure out that there was and continues to be nothing wrong with me. Yeah, I couldn't figure out how to say no to a drink. But that didn't mean I should stop *trying* to learn. And so, as soon as I called my roommate, found a bail bondsman, and got my ass out of County Holding, I set about teaching myself to say no. In many ways, it was a lot like wearing an emotional scarlet A on my chest—but while Hester Prynne's A meant *Adultress*, mine meant *Abuser*. And I didn't bother putting it on my actual clothes—just because other people couldn't see it didn't mean I didn't wear my A with stoic pride.

I'd always hated feeling lonely—I had never realized how much my social drinking was to avoid that feeling.

I started hanging out at bars less. *Much* less. Instead of going out for a beer after work with friends, I would quietly slip out the back door and head home. When I did decide to go out, I paid attention to how much I drank. That was something I'd literally never done before. I also spent more time alone. I'd always hated feeling lonely—I had never realized how much my social drinking was to avoid that feeling. Plus, it wasn't until I ended up in a scary and life-changing situation that I realized I needed to learn a little thing called self-control.

To this day, I remain in a process of understanding how to handle the presence of alcohol. I spent years being too embarrassed to actually attribute the word *alcoholic* with my own behavior. But now I'm more comfortable acknowledging the presence of alcoholic tendencies in my own life. And it's made me acknowledge that loneliness isn't the world's best reason to pick up a drink.

These days I try to challenge myself to feel lonely, to really absorb it as an emotional experience. I still don't really like it. And it's still very hard to resist a drink when I'm in a situation that makes me feel uncomfortable. To this day, I have very intentional conversations with myself, and I ask myself questions I would never have thought to ask myself before my DWI. And since I started wearing my scarlet A, the importance of my yoga practice has come into much more vivid color. Not necessarily the asana part, but the other limbs of the path that are too oft forgotten—at the very least satya, the yama of truthfulness (page 36), is what requires that I ask these questions of myself.

LESSON LEARNED

Basically, I'm really fucking grateful that Mr. Nice Cop found me in that intersection—I needed a wake-up call. Instead of going out to a bar, I started practicing a very specific sequence of core-centric yoga poses that worked my abs while also distracting me from my stress. This is that sequence—it will get your body fired up with lots of sweat, and if you do several repetitions with a deep ujjayi breath (page 65), I guarantee the intensity of the sequencing will ease your weary mind.

I NEED TO CHILL

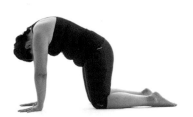

1. CAT/COW POSE (PAGE 114)

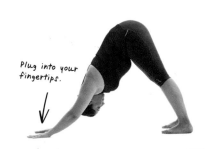

Plug into your fingertips.

4. DOWNWARD-FACING DOG (PAGE 80)

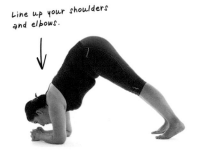

Line up your shoulders and elbows.

5. DOLPHIN POSE (PAGE 99)

THE F OUT

Stack your wrist and shoulder joints.

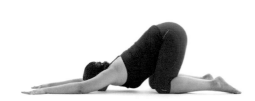

2. EXTENDED PUPPY DOG POSE (PAGE 115)

3. HIGH PLANK (PAGE 94)

Take a vinyaasa (page 167) and repeat.

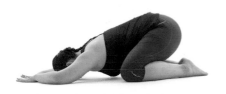

6. CHILD'S POSE (PAGE 124)

ONE IS THE MAGIC NUMBER

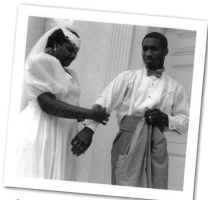

The Afro-American Ozzy and Harriet on their wedding day.

My alcohol problem didn't materialize out of thin air; I think it was rooted in an inability to accept self-love. In many ways, self-love has been the great pursuit of my life. Popular wisdom would say that loving yourself is a matter of reminding yourself, "I'm beautiful! I'm perfect!" about ten million times over and over until you believe it. But I've never found the "I'm beautiful!" method to be very effective. If I'm being *truly* honest with myself, I think my own self-love vacuum has had more to do with loneliness than anything else.

I've always despised loneliness. In fact, I've gone out of my way to flat-out avoid it on more than one occasion. You probably know all the tricks: Have you ever refused to eat alone in a restaurant, and maybe called up a friend at the last minute just so you don't have to be seen alone in public? Or maybe you've stayed home instead of attending a potentially fun party out of fear of standing alone among strangers? Yeah. Me too.

No one ever wants to admit their "weaknesses," but I think I've been trying to fend off loneliness from the moment I was pushed out of Tangela's womb. My aversion to loneliness crops up in weird ways and at inconvenient times. It doesn't wait solely for the moments when I'm alone—often, I notice it the most when I'm surrounded by other people.

Over the years, I've developed an endless stream of (ultimately futile) tactics to avoid acknowledging my loneliness: epic shopping binges, Hemingway-style drunken benders, forest-fire-level marijuana blazes, Dionysian food gorges.

But my addiction to serial monogamy is probably my most significant loneliness-fighting vice. When I was a little femme, I always assumed I would get married and have a family. Perhaps it's because I was raised to be a good little Bahá'í girl? A Good Little Bahá'í Girl considers service to God, family, and the world at large to be the pinnacle of her value system. And, as the quintessential Good Little Bahá'í Girl, I always assumed I would get married and have a family. A solid, functioning nuclear family is kind of like the prized jewel of the Bahá'í lifestyle—families are considered central to the progression of the Bahá'í faith, and believers are strongly encouraged to practice staunch abstinence until marriage. Once married, Bahá'í are encouraged to breed heavily, producing a herd of well-behaved, effortlessly sober, morally pacifistic do-gooders.

Because of Jesse and Tangela's commitment to embodying the spirit of an Afro-American Ozzy and Harriet, I was raised in a bubble of mutual respect, love, and seemingly faithful support. From a young age, I idolized my parents' relationship and I prayed to anyone within spiritual hearing range for my personal variation of their happiness—a loving partner of my very own with whom I would share a life and a family. Coming out as a lesbian at the age of seventeen and coming out again as queer in my early twenties did nothing to dampen this pursuit. I held a fantasy of a loving wife and adopted babies at the epicenter of happiness goals.

I believed this commitment to a devoted partner would fulfill, sustain, and provide me with a life purpose. In essence, it would help establish and confirm my identity. Second only to college matriculation, I considered the pursuit of a permanent romantic costar to be one of my primary goals in life. And so, from the moment I was socialized with other kids my age, I became very interested in rounding out my sense of self through a loving relationship with another person.

I've always allowed my long-term partners to become not just my loves, but crucial backbones of my identity. Instead of telling myself "I love you," I developed an addiction to hearing it *only* when uttered from the lips of other people. And on this lonely road, it's always been much easier for me to tell other people "I love you!" as opposed to looking in the mirror and saying "I love you" to myself.

The dissolution of the major "loves of my life" were dramatic and painful, but also extremely run-of-the-mill—I bet you're hiding a similar closet of relationship skeletons. However, each of these heartbreaks has helped my yoga practice to grow, particularly when it comes to understanding the Yama of Brahmacharya—aka "chastity."

Let me be clear. I'm not talking about actual chastity—the no-sex-ever kind. It's more like an emotional chastity. Here's how I see it: When we engage in sexual relations with other people, we enter into one of the most intimate of human connections; but these encounters should not define us. For me, chastity is about trying not to use sex and the love of others as a path toward self-love. So these days, I try to spend more time alone than with other people. The result is that I've unwrapped a whole new method of self-love. It's made me capable of standing alone, as one solitary, strong individual, without relying on the support of one specific other being. In that way, Brahmacharya has allowed me to release a slew of internal demons.

It's easy to love yourself when someone else has declared their love for you. But there's an unmistakable power in establishing self-love all by your lonesome. This can be a scary thing to do. It means spending more time alone than with lovers, family, and friends. It means experiencing true loneliness. Because only when we're alone are we given a front-row seat to the magic of our own existence.

LESSONS LEARNED

When it comes to asana practice, being alone on the yoga mat is frightening for many of us, because it's an intense reminder of what it feels like to be lonely. Some of us refuse to be totally alone on our mats, and we prefer the company of our teachers and fellow students to help block out the corresponding sensations of loneliness. But I think that the time we spend alone on our mats is crucial on more than just one level. We are able to fully focus our attention and our *intention*, so that we are not distracted by the needs, wants, and opinions of others. In my own life, the time I've spent alone on my yoga mat has become more of an asset than anything else.

The following sequence, which incorporates a variety of different yoga props and bodily modifications, is all about self-love. In my humble opinion, no vigorous vinyasa-style yoga practice is complete without a series of cooling, restorative postures to round out your body conditioning. This sequence can stand by its lonesome or it can be paired with other sequences. Give yourself free rein to make the poses as restorative as you'd like by using the recommended props. Think of this sequence as a loving squeeze from the universe—the singular purpose is to simply make your body feel good.

I NEED TO

Use as a stand-alone sequence, or begin with either I Want to Stand Strong (page 166), I Need to Feel Balanced (page 176), I Want to See the World from Another Angle (page 186), or I Need to Release Fear (page 200).

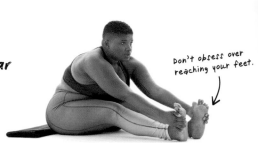

Don't obsess over reaching your feet.

1. SEATED FORWARD BEND (PAGE 125)

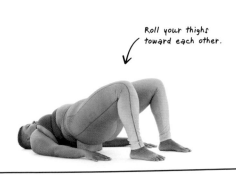

Roll your thighs toward each other.

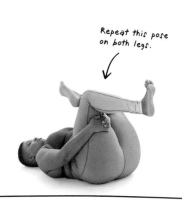

Repeat this pose on both legs.

4. BRIDGE (PAGE 122)

5. THREAD THE NEEDLE (PAGE 111)

LOVE MYSELF

Relax your shoulders.

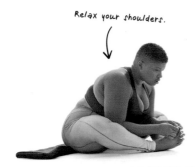

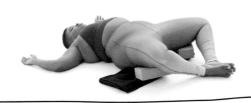

2. BOUND ANGLE (PAGE 126)

3. RECLINED BOUND ANGLE (PAGE 128)

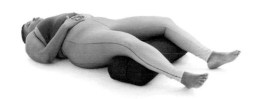

6. CORPSE (PAGE 130)

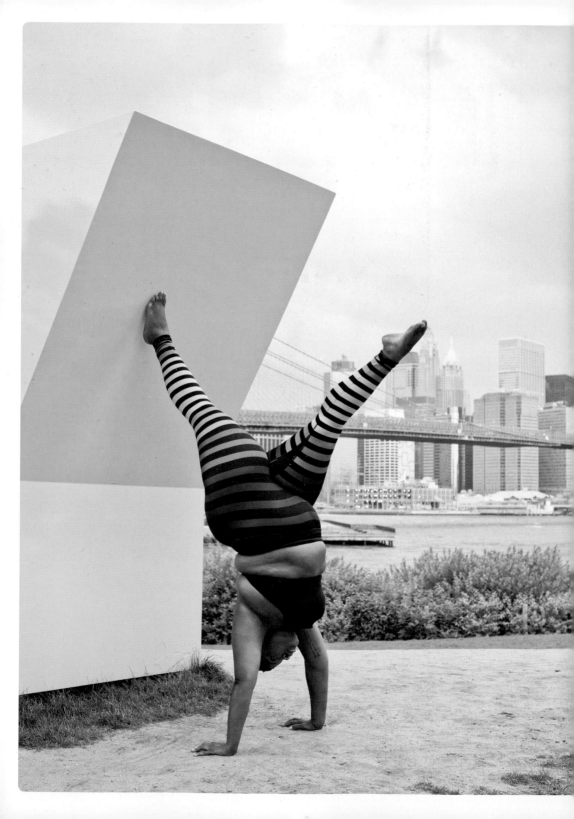

PART 5

Is It Really That Simple?

Every day of my monthlong yoga teacher training (YTT for short), at least one trainee would dissolve into tears over some deep-seated and long-ignored emotional trauma.

While I considered myself open to the more touchy-feely aspects of the yogic experience, all of the spontaneous emotional outbursts weirded me out. After all, I was raised to be a strong black woman—a take-shit-from-nobody, support-my-family-against-all-odds, fight-to-the-death strong black woman. And strong black women DO NOT cry. The only situations in which we're allowed to cry are on our wedding day, at family funerals, and during childbirth. Other than that, the general mentality is "suck it up and get back to work, bitch." That, on top of having been bullied as an adolescent, made me the master of my emotions, and I prided myself on how infrequently I needed to cry (usually only once every few months or so).

One day during YTT, while practicing a series of partner yoga exercises requiring us to lean on/bear weight on each other, I was paired with Katie, a petite(ish) blond and heavily tattooed yoga angel. I was intimidated by the idea of working with Katie because her body was so dramatically smaller than my own. Because I've been conditioned to see my size as a problem, I compulsively apologized to her throughout the practice—every movement we made together elicited an audible and meek "sorry!" from yours truly.

Eventually, Katie stopped moving and looked me dead in the eye. "You know," she said, with a tone as sweet as cherry pie, "you don't have to apologize for everything."

I stopped what I was doing and let out a little laugh and my trademark grin, a smile I honed back in my pageant days. "I know," I said, smiling and shrugging my shoulders. "I guess I'm just apologizing for existing." Katie cocked her eyebrow at me and got back into position for our practice. I, on the other hand, was stopped dead in my tracks.

I was shocked. I couldn't recall ever thinking something so pathetic about myself. And the words had slipped out effortlessly, as though they'd always been on the edge of my tongue.

"I'M APOLOGIZING FOR EXISTING??" I screamed at myself. How the FUCK could I actually think something like that, let alone SAY IT OUT LOUD? But in that moment, I knew that I meant it.

I began to sob. I tried to keep the sound under control—I was, after all, literally practicing yoga with another human being, in a room full of people. But Katie (bless her) didn't mention it. Like I said, EVERYONE WAS CRYING DURING YTT and now that it was my turn, I couldn't stop. I cried for the rest of the practice. I cried all throughout Savasana. I cried in my car after class while everyone else drove home for the night. I cried as I drove back to my house. I cried until I fell asleep that night.

It was one of the saddest and darkest self-realizations I've ever made. It hit me to my core. But would I have ever reached that point if I hadn't practiced yoga? Sure, I might've continued walking around in my daily life misdiagnosing my internal unhappiness. And it's not like I'm magically a different person—even to this day, I compulsively apologize for things all the time. I can't really help it—it's the plight of the Southern woman in many ways. But now that I've actually acknowledged the problem, I can work toward eliminating it from my being.

> **The work doesn't really start or end on a yoga mat.**

This is the eight-limbed path in action. The work doesn't really start or end on a yoga mat. The only purpose of asana is to build heat and focus so we can draw conclusions about ourselves and the world at large. That's the journey that I want for you. That's the yoga journey you deserve. Not an exercise regimen.

When you close this book and roll out a yoga mat, you may find that some of the steps I've outlined here are much more difficult than you expected. You may find that maintaining an even, steady ujjayi breath is much harder than it seems. You may even find that some of the asana that look totally doable in earlier pages feel impossible in real life. And, inevitably, it's likely that your fledgling eight-limbed path yoga practice will provoke noisy and obtrusive emotions that you would have rather kept quiet.

If for nothing else, these reactions are the reason you should come to your mat. I cannot stress this enough: Allow your yoga practice to be arduous and difficult, without complaint. Don't prevent your outpouring of emotion. Don't resist the trembles. Continue coming to your mat, even when something makes you feel uncomfortable.

I can only speak for myself, but the mere act of sitting quietly can be enough to flare up a series of internal alarms. Still, I never regret surrendering myself to the practice. And the time I've spent sitting all by my lonesome, staring intently within myself, has been the most worthwhile time I've spent while alive on this planet.

At the end of the day, we all struggle with emotional, physical, and spiritual turmoil. This struggle is our great unifier. And if we all deal with the same struggles, yoga is the equalizing influence that can calm all of our lives. Yoga is for everyone, and body shape/size/color is *completely* irrelevant. Whatever your shape, shade, whatever baggage you're carrying around with you, put it down and get on the mat. Find a place for yoga in your life today.

XOXO,
Jessamyn

INDEX

ACKNOWLEDGMENTS

Thank you, Maisie—so much would be shitty without you.

To Jane, Jessy, and Miriam—thanks for standing by my side, cracking the whip, and making sure no one throws a knife in my back.

To Christine, Jonathan, Steph, Anne, Becky, Laura, Chrissie, Jac, Charlie, Angela, Amanda, and Annie—you're truly the unsung heroes of this project. Thanks for sharing your unique gifts with me.

To Tangela, Jesse, Gabriel—thanks for always accepting me exactly as I am.

To Tiriah, Marvella, Tracy, EmmaLou, and Jemma—thanks for being the embodiment of strength and power.

To Betty B., who told me to write "Tabor City Funerals"—you were right. Thank you.

To Samantha, Dallas, and James—thank you for being my home.

To my Durham squad—thanks for filling my heart with joy and always offering yourselves up as yoga guinea pigs. Furthermore, thanks for helping this Greensboro party femme get her shit together.

To the teachers who changed my life: Kimberley, Stephanie, Michael, Joe, Libby, Shala, Sierra, Ryan, Ruth, and Jane Anne—you've touched my heart and my yoga practice forever.

To my YTT trainee family—"I Am Thine, In Mine Myself, Wahe Guru."

To Anna Guest-Jelley, Dianne Bondy, Amber Karnes, and Valerie Sagun—thank you for lighting my fire.

To Kathryn Budig, Amy Ippoliti, Tara Judelle, Giselle Mari, Elena Brower, and Meghan Currie—thank you for pouring lighter fluid on my fire.

To Trudi Swenk, Bruce Swenk, and Alison Hinks—thank you for showing me what a body-positive yoga environment can look like in action.

To everyone who bullied me in middle school—thank you for making me stronger.

And to everyone who asked me to write this book—thank you for being my inspiration.